An Atlas of
BACK PAIN

THE ENCYCLOPEDIA OF VISUAL MEDICINE SERIES

An Atlas of
BACK PAIN

Scott D. Haldeman

DC, MD, PhD, FRCP(C), FCCS(C)

Clinical Professor, Department of Neurology
University of California, Irvine, California, USA

William H. Kirkaldy-Willis

MA, MD, LLD(Hon), FRCS(E and C), FACS, FICC(Hon)

Emeritus Professor and Head, Department of Orthopedic Surgery,
University of Saskatchewan College of Medicine, Saskatoon, Saskatchewan, Canada

Thomas N. Bernard, Jr

MD

Clinical Assistant Professor, Department of Orthopedic Surgery
Tulane University School of Medicine, New Orleans, Louisiana, USA

The Parthenon Publishing Group
International Publishers in Medicine, Science & Technology

A CRC PRESS COMPANY
BOCA RATON   LONDON   NEW YORK   WASHINGTON, D.C.

Published in the USA by
The Parthenon Publishing Group
345 Park Avenue South, 10th Floor
New York
NY 10010
USA

Published in the UK by
The Parthenon Publishing Group
23–25 Blades Court
Deodar Road
London SW15 2NU
UK

Copyright © 2002 The Parthenon Publishing Group

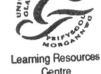

Library of Congress Cataloging-in-Publication Data
Haldeman, Scott.
  An atlas of back pain / Scott Haldeman, William H. Kirkaldy-Willis, Thomas N.
Bernard, Jr.
    p. ; cm. -- (The encyclopedia of visual medicine series)
  Includes bibliographical references and index.
  ISBN 1-84214-076-0 (alk. paper)
    1. Backache--Atlases. I. Title: Back pain. II. Kirkaldy-Willis, W. H. III. Bernard,
Thomas N. IV. Title. V. Series.
    [DNLM: 1. Back Pain--etiology--Atlases. 2. Back Pain--diagnosis--Atlases. 3. Spinal
Diseases--pathology--Atlases. WE 17 H159a 2002]
  RD771.B217H354 2002
  617.5'64'00222--dc21   2001056029

British Library Cataloguing in Publication Data
Haldeman, Scott
  An atlas of back pain. - (The encyclopedia of visual medicine series)
  1. Backache
  I. Title II. Kirkaldy-Willis, W. H. III. Bernard, Thomas N.
  617.5'64

ISBN 1-84214-076-0

First published in 2002

Composition by The Parthenon Publishing Group
Color reproduction by Graphic Reproductions, UK
Printed and bound by T. G. Hostench S.A., Spain

Contents

Preface

There are few greater challenges to clinicians than the diagnosis and treatment of patients with back pain. The process of making such a diagnosis requires an understanding of the complex anatomy and physiology of the spine and the ability to differentiate between structural, functional, congenital and pathological conditions that can occur in the spine and potentially cause or impact upon the symptoms of back pain and decreased functional capacity. The ability to examine and treat patients with back pain is dependent on the ability of a clinician to visualize changes that can occur in the normal structure and function of the spine that may result in pain, and to assess the effect of the social, occupational and emotional factors that may impact upon the manner in which a patient responds to pain.

This *Atlas of Back Pain* is an effort to help the clinician in the visualization of the spine by defining normal and abnormal spinal anatomy and physiology. This will be attempted by means of diagrams, anatomical and pathological slides as well as the presentation of imaging and physiological tests that are available to the clinician and which can be used to assist in the diagnosis of patients with back pain.

In order to achieve this goal, it was felt appropriate to make this text a team effort, since no one specialty or area of expertise has been found able to adequately present the complex issues associated with back pain. The pathological slides accumulated over 30 years by one of the authors (W.H. Kirkaldy-Willis) have been supplemented with imaging studies from a very busy orthopedic practice (T.N. Bernard) and experience in clinical and experimental neurophysiology (S. Haldeman) so as to present a comprehensive picture of the factors which should be considered in evaluating patients with back pain. This text is truly a combination of the experience and expertise of the three authors.

Acknowledgements

We appreciate the permission received from Churchill Livingstone (Saunders) Press to republish figures of pathology from *Managing Low Back Pain*, 4th edition, edited by W.H. Kirkaldy-Willis and T.N. Bernard Jr.

We acknowledge permission from Dr R.R. Cooper (Iowa City) to publish his electron microscope figures of 'Regeneration of skeletal muscle in the cat' included in this text.

We thank Dr J.D. Cassidy, Dr K. Yong Hing, Dr J. Reilly and Mr J. Junor for their help in obtaining, preparing and photographing pathological specimens used in this Atlas.

We are indebted to Dr D.B. Allbrook and Dr W. de C. Baker for their help with the section on Muscle repair.

1

Introduction

Back pain, like tooth decay and the common cold, is an affliction that affects a substantial proportion, if not the entire population, at some point in their lives. Nobody is immune to this condition nor its potential disability which does not discriminate by gender, age, race or culture. It has become one of the leading causes of disability in our society and the cost of treatment has been increasing progressively each year, without any obvious effect on the frequency and severity of the condition. The search for a cure and the elimination of back pain does not appear to be a viable option at this point in our understanding of back pain. A reasonable goal, however, is to improve the ability of clinicians to determine the cause of back pain in a substantial proportion of patients, to identify conditions likely to lead to serious disability if not treated promptly, to reduce the symptoms of back pain, to increase functional capacity and to reduce the likelihood of recurrences.

EPIDEMIOLOGY

The prevalence of back pain in the adult population varies with age. There are a number of surveys in multiple countries that reveal a point-prevalence of 17–30%, a 1-month prevalence of 19–43% and a lifetime prevalence of 60–80%. The likelihood that an individual will recall on survey that they have experienced back pain in their lifetime reaches 80% by the age of 60 years, and there is some evidence that the remaining 20% have simply forgotten prior episodes of back pain or considered such episodes as a natural part of life and not worth reporting. At the age of 40 years, the prevalence is slightly higher in women, while, after the age of 50, it is slightly higher

in men. The majority of these episodes of back pain are mild and short-lived and have very little impact on daily life. Recurrences are common and one survey found that up to 14% of the adult population had an episode of back pain each year that lasted 30 days or longer and at some point interfered with sleep, routine activities or work. Approximately 1% of the population is permanently disabled by back pain at any given point, with another 1–2% temporarily disabled from their normal occupation. Children and adolescents are not immune from back pain. Surveys reveal that approximately 5% of all children have a history of back pain that interferes with activity, with 27% reporting back pain at some time.

Figure 1.1 The prevalence rates for low back pain in the general population by age

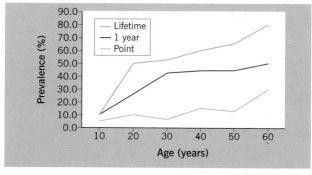

The lifetime prevalence represents the report of symptoms having occurred at any time prior to the date of enquiry or survey. The 1-year prevalence represents the likelihood that a person will report an episode of pain in the year before an enquiry. Point-prevalence is the likelihood on survey of a person reporting pain at the time of the enquiry. Adapted from references 1–3 with permission

WORK-RELATED BACK PAIN

Back injuries make up one-third of all work-related injuries or almost one million claims in the United States each year. Approximately 150 million work-days are lost each year, affecting 17% of all American workers. Half of the lost workdays are taken by 15% of this population, usually with prolonged periods of time loss, while the other 50% of lost work days are for periods of less than 1 week. The incidence rates for work-related back injuries vary, depending on the type of work performed. The factors that increase the likelihood of back injury are repetitive heavy lifting, prolonged bending and twisting, repetitive heavy pushing and pulling activities and long periods of vibration exposure. Work that requires minimal physically strenuous activity, such as the finance, insurance and service industries, has the lowest back injury rates, whereas work requiring repetitive and strenuous activity such as construction, mining and forestry has the highest injury rates.

PATHOLOGY AND BACK PAIN

There is a strong inclination on the part of clinicians and patients suffering from back pain, especially if it is associated with disability, to relate the symptoms of pain to pathological changes in spinal tissues. For this reason, there is a tendency to look for anatomi-cal abnormalities to explain the presence of pain, by ordering X-rays, computerized tomography (CT) or magnetic resonance imaging (MRI) studies. It is tempting to point to changes in anatomical structure seen on these studies as the cause of the symptoms. Unfortunately, the assumption that the lesion seen on these studies is the cause of the pain is not always valid. Degenerative changes occur in virtually all patients as part of the normal aging process. At age 20, degenerative changes are noted on X-ray and MRI in less than 10% of the population. By age 40, such changes are seen in 50% of the asymptomatic population and, by age 60, this number reaches over 90%. Disc and joint pathology is noted in 100% of autopsies of persons over the age of 50. These changes can affect multiple levels of the spine and can be severe in the absence of symptoms.

Pathology in the intervertebral disc can also exist in the absence of symptoms. Disc protrusion or herniation can be found in 30–50% of the population in the absence of symptoms. Even large and dramatic disc herniations and extrusions can be found in asymptomatic individuals. Changes in the intervertebral disc seen on discography, including fissures and radial tears, have recently been found to exist in patients without back pain. It is, therefore, not possible to interpret pathology seen on imaging studies as the origin of a person's back pain without looking for other contributing factors or clinical findings.

Figure 1.2 The incidence of work-related back pain by industry

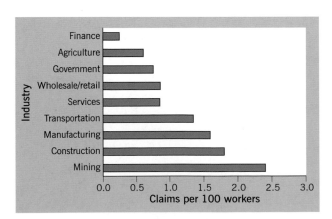

The more physically stressful and demanding the occupation, the greater the likelihood of disability due to back pain. Adapted from reference 4 with permission

Figure 1.3 The incidence of pathology in the normal population

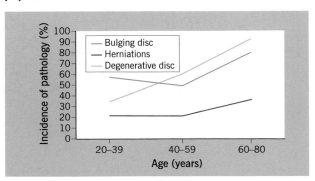

Disc herniations, disc bulging and degenerative changes are very common in the asymptomatic population. Most individuals can anticipate pathological changes on MRI, CT scan or radiographs, even in the absence of symptoms. Under certain circumstances, these changes can become symptomatic. Adapted from reference 5, with permission

PHYSIOLOGY OF BACK PAIN

There are a number of factors that have been implicated in the genesis of back pain and disability that can be used to determine whether a pathological process seen on imaging studies is associated with symptoms experienced by a patient. Certain of these factors are based on epidemiological studies, while others are based on clinical findings and physiological tests.

Pain in any structure requires the release of inflammatory agents that stimulate pain receptors and generate a nociceptive response in the tissue. The spine is unique in that it has multiple structures that are innervated by pain fibers. Inflammation of the posterior joints of the spine, the intervertebral disc, the ligaments and muscles, meninges and nerve roots have all been associated with back pain. These tissues respond to injury by releasing a number of chemical agents that include bradykinin, prostaglandins and leukotrienes. These chemical agents activate nerve endings and generate nerve impulses that travel to the spinal cord. The nociceptive nerves, in turn, release neuropeptides, the most prominent of which is substance P. These neuropeptides act on blood vessels, causing extravasation, and stimulate mast cells to release histamine and dilate blood vessels. The mast cells also release leukotrienes and other inflammatory chemicals that attract polymorphonuclear leukocytes and monocytes. These processes result in the classic findings of inflammation with tissue swelling, vascular congestion and further stimulation of painful nerve endings.

The pain impulses generated from injured and inflamed spinal tissues are transmitted via nerve fibers that travel through the anterior (from nerves innervating the extremities) and posterior (from the dorsal musculature) primary divisions of the spinal nerves and through the posterior nerve roots and the dorsal root ganglia to the spinal cord, where they make connections with ascending fibers that transmit the pain sensation to the brain. The spinal cord and brain have developed a mechanism of modifying the pain impulses coming from spinal tissues. At the level of the spinal cord , the pain impulses converge on neurons that also receive input from other sensory receptors. This results in changes in the degree of pain sensation that is transmitted to the brain through a process commonly referred to as the 'gate control' system. The pain impulses are modified further through a complex process that occurs at multiple levels of the central nervous system. The brain releases chemical agents in response to pain known as endorphins. These function as natural analgesics. The brain can also block or enhance the pain response by means of descending serotonergic modulating pathways that impact with pain

Figure 1.4 Neurophysiology of spinal pain

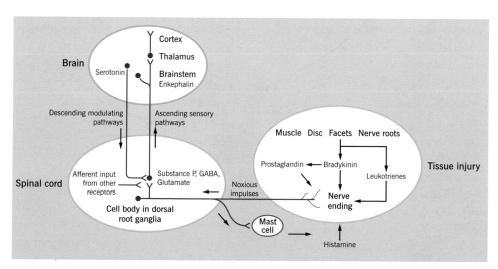

A simplified diagram of neurophysiological pathways and a few of the neurotransmitters responsible for spinal pain. Injury to the spinal tissues results in the release of inflammatory agents which stimulate nerve endings. Impulses travel to the spinal cord and connect to neurons which send impulses to the brain via the brainstem. There is a spinal cord-modulating system in the spinal cord which interacts with other afferent input and descending modulating pathways from the periaqueductal gray matter and other brainstem nuclei

Figure 1.5 A model for spinal disability

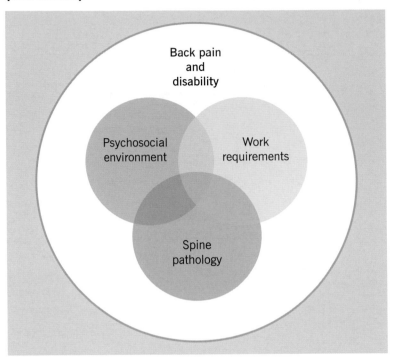

This model is one manner of visualizing the interaction of spine pathology, work requirements and psychosocial factors in the genesis of back pain and its resulting disability

sensations both centrally and at the spinal cord level. The latter mechanism is felt to be responsible for the strong impact of psychosocial factors on the response to pain and the disability associated with back pain. The pain centers in the spinal cord and brain can also change through a process known as plasticity which may explain the observation that many patients develop chronic pain that is more widespread than the pathological lesion and continues after the resolution of the peripheral inflammatory process.

APPROACHING THE PATIENT WITH BACK PAIN

The factors that determine the degree of back pain, and especially the amount of disability associated with the pain, are therefore the result of multiple factors. Structural pathology sets the stage and is the origin of the painful stimulus. The natural healing process, in most situations, results in the resolution of back pain within relatively short periods. Physical stress placed on the back through work and leisure activities may slow the healing process or irritate spinal pathology such as degenerative changes or disc protrusion. It is, however, the psychosocial situation

of the patient that determines the level of discomfort and the response of a patient to the painful stimulus. The patient's psychological state, level of satisfaction with work and personal life as well as his/her social and spiritual life may impact upon the central modulation system in the brain and modify the response to pain.

In this volume, a great deal of emphasis is placed on visualization of spinal lesions that can result in spinal pain. To rely on anatomical changes to determine the cause of back pain can, however, be very misleading to the clinician through the mechanisms described above. There are other examples in science that can be used as a model for looking at spinal pain. The Danish pioneer of quantum physics, Niels Bohr, claimed that science does not adequately explain the way the world is but rather only the way we, as observers, *interact* with this world. Early in the last century, it was discovered that light could be explained in terms of either waves or particles, depending on the type of experiment that was set up by the observer. Bohr postulated that it was the *interaction* between the scientist, as the observer, and the phenomenon being studied, in this case light, that was important. The same thing can be said for the clinician approaching a patient with back pain. The conclusions reached by the clinician regarding the etiology of back pain in a specific case are often dependent on the interaction between the patient and the clinician and the training and experience brought to the decision-making process by both individuals.

There are other ways of looking at back pain. Chaos theory postulates that there is a delicate balance between disorder and order. The origin of the universe is generally explained by the 'Big Bang' theory which states that, in the beginning, there was total disorder which was followed by the gradual imposition of order through the creation of galaxies, stars and planets. This process is perceived as occurring through a delicate balance between the forces of gravity and the effects of the initial explosion. This process emphasizes that small changes at the beginning of a process or reaction can result in large changes over time. If one applies this analogy to the interaction between patients with back pain and their physicians, the outcome of treatment can be perceived as being impacted upon by a number of beneficial influences or 'little nudges' and harmful attitudes or 'little ripples' (Table 1). The patient's symptoms can be positively impacted through such processes as listening, caring, laughter, explanation, encouragement, attention to detail and even prayer and negatively impacted by fear, anxiety, anger, uncertainty, boredom and haste. The manner in which a physician uses these nudges and helps the patient avoid the ripples can have a large effect on the impact of back pain on the patient's life. The most accurate diagnosis possible is dependent on accurately observing and listening to the patient, the physical examination and the results of all testing in combination with the intuition that is gained from experience from treating multiple similar patients.

The fine balance between different factors impacting on back pain can be illustrated by a few simple examples.

Example 1

A 50-year-old woman presented to her doctor with symptoms and signs of a disc herniation confirmed by CT scan. She was the owner of a small cattle range and was worried about the condition of her animals. She underwent surgery to correct the disc herniation but her convalescence was prolonged for no apparent reason. After several months, the condition of her cattle herd improved and, at the same time, the patient's symptoms improved. This raises the question as to the link between the patient's symptoms, the disc herniation and the condition of her cattle.

Example 2

A 45-year-old gentleman in a position with a responsible insurance company presented to his doctor with symptoms and signs of severe L4–5 instability confirmed by stress X-rays. The patient underwent a posterolateral fusion. At 3 months, the fusion was solid but the patient's symptoms did not improve. Further questioning revealed that he felt stressed and was unhappy in his work. At 6 months, he became symptom-free without further treatment. The only evident change in his status was the resolution of his difficulties at work.

Example 3

A 35-year-old gentleman with a wife and two small children was admitted to the hospital on an emergency basis with suspected cauda equina syndrome. A psychotherapist assigned to the case discovered that the patient found the presence of his mother-in-law intolerable. Arrangements were made for the mother-in-law to live elsewhere and the patient made an uneventful recovery without the necessity of surgery.

Table 1 Beneficial influences (nudges) and harmful influences (ripples) which impact on the outcome of treament for back pain

Harmful influences	Beneficial influences
Fear	Listening and caring
Anxiety	Laughter
Anger	Explanation
Uncertainty	Encouragement
Boredom	Attention
Haste	Prayer

REFERENCES

1. Andersson GBJ. The epidemiology of spinal disorders. In Frymoyer JW, ed. *The Adult Spine, Principles and Practice*, 2nd edn. Philadelphia: Lippincott-Raven, 1997

2. Burton AK, Clarke RD, McClune TD, Tillotson KM. The natural history of low back pain in adolescents. *Spine* 1996;21:2323–8

3. Taimela S, Kujala UM, Salminem JJ, Viljanen T. The prevalence of low back pain among children and adolescents. A nationwide, cohort-based questionnaire survey in Finland. *Spine* 1997;22:1132–6

4. Frymoyer JW, ed. *The Adult Spine. Principles and Practice*, 2nd edn. Philadelphia: Lippincott-Raven, 1997

5. Boden S, Davis DO, Dina TS, Patronas NJ, Wiesel SW. Abnormal magnetic-resonance scans of the lumbar spine in asymptomatic subjects. *J Bone Joint Surg* 1990;72-A(3):403–8

6. Hartvigsen J, Bakketeig LS, Leboeuf-Y de C, Engberg M, Lauritzen T. The association between physical workload and low back pain clouded by the "healthy worker" effect. *Spine* 2001;26:1788–93

7. Kuslich SD, Ulstrom CL, Michael CJ. The tissue origin of low back pain and sciatica: a report of pain response to tissue stimulation during operations on the lumbar spine using local anesthesia. *Orthop Clin N Am* 1991;22:181

8. Bigos SJ, Battie MC. Risk factors for industrial back problems. *Semin Spine Surg* 1992;4:2

9. Kelsey J, Golden A. Occupational and workplace factors associated with low back pain. *Spine* 1987; 2:7

10. Sanderson PL, Todd BD, Holt GR, *et al.* Compensation, work status, and disability in low back pain patients. *Spine* 1995;20:554

11. Haldeman S, Shouka S, Robboy S. Computerized tomography, electrodiagnosis and clinical findings in chronic worker's compensation patients with back and leg pain. *Spine* 1988; 3:345–50

2

Normal spinal anatomy and physiology

The spine is one of the most complex structures in the body. It is a structure that includes bones, muscles, ligaments, nerves and blood vessels as well as diarthrodial joints. In addition, the structures that make up the spine include the intervertebral discs, the nerve roots and dorsal root ganglia, the spinal cord and the dura mater with its spaces filled with cerebrospinal fluid. Each of these structures has unique responses to trauma, aging and activity.

THE BONY VERTEBRAE

Each of the bony elements of the back consist of a heavy kidney-shaped bony structure known as the vertebral body, a horseshoe-shaped vertebral arch made up of a lamina, pedicles and seven protruding processes. The pedicle attaches to the superior half of the vertebral body and extends backwards to the articular pillar. The articular pillar extends rostrally and caudally to form the superior and inferior facet joints. The transverse processes extend laterally from the posterior aspect of the articular pillar where it connects to a flat broad bony lamina. The laminae extend posteriorly from the left and right articular pillars and join to form the spinous process. Two adjacent vertebrae connect with each other by means of the facet joints on either side. This leaves a space between the bodies of the vertebrae which is filled with the intervertebral disc. The intervertebral foramen for the exiting nerve root is formed by the space between the adjacent pedicles, facet joints and the vertebral body and disc. The integrity of the nerve root canal is therefore dependent on the integrity of the facet joints, the articular pillars, the vertebral body endplates and the intervertebral disc.

The bony vertebrae can be visualized on standard radiographs and on CT scan using X-radiation. The bones can also be visualized on MRI, although with not quite the same definition. The metabolism of the bony vertebra can be visualized by means of a technetium bone scan.

Figure 2.1 Superior view of an isolated lumbar vertebra

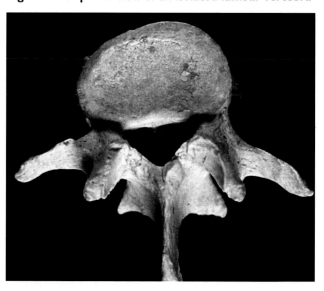

This view demonstrates the two posterior facets and the vertebral body endplate where the disc attaches. The facets and the disc make up the 'three-joint complex' of the spinal motion segment. The body of the vertebra is connected to the articular pillars by the pedicles. The superior and inferior articular facets extend from the articular pillars to connect with the corresponding facets of the vertebrae above and below, to make up the posterior facets. The lateral transverse processes and the posterior spinous process form the attachments for paraspinal ligaments and muscles. Courtesy Churchill-Livingstone (Saunders) Press

THE INTERVERTEBRAL DISC

The intervertebral disc is made up of an outer annulus fibrosis and a central nucleus pulposus. It is attached to the vertebral bodies above and below the disc by the superior and inferior endplates. The nucleus pulposus is a gel-like substance made up of a meshwork of collagen fibrils suspended in a mucopolysaccharide base. It has a high water content in young individuals, which gradually diminishes with degenerative changes and with the natural aging process. The annulus fibrosis is made up of a series of concentric fibrocartilaginous lamellae which run at an oblique angle of about 30° orientation to the plane of the disc. The fibers of adjacent lamellae have similar arrangements, but run in opposite directions. The fibers of the outer annulus lamella attach to the vertebral body and mingle with the periosteal fibers. The fibrocartilaginous endplates are made up of hyaline cartilage and attach to the subchondral bone plate of the vertebral bodies. There are multiple small vascular perforations in the endplate, which allow nutrition to pass to the disc.

The intervertebral disc is not seen on standard X-ray, but can be visualized by means of MRI scan and CT scan. The integrity of the inner aspects of the disc is best visualized by injecting a radio-opaque agent into the disc. This material disperses within the nucleus and can be visualized radiologically as a discogram.

Figure 2.2 Lateral view of the L3 and L4 vertebrae

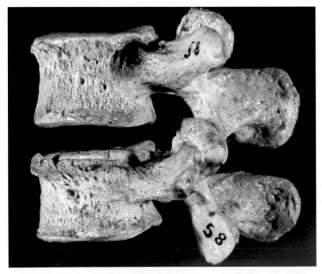

This projection demonstrates the manner in which the facets join. The space between the vertebral bodies is the location of the cartilaginous intervertebral disc. Courtesy Churchill-Livingstone (Saunders) Press

THE POSTERIOR FACETS

The facet joints connect the superior facet of a vertebra to the inferior facet of the adjacent vertebra on each side and are typical synovial joints. The articular surfaces are made of hyaline cartilage which is thicker in the center of the facet and thinner at the edges. A circumferential fibrous capsule, which is continuous with the ligamentum flavum ventrally, joins the two facet surfaces. Fibroadipose vascular tissue extends into the joint space from the capsule, particularly at the proximal and distal poles. This tissue has been referred to as a meniscoid which can become entrapped between the facets.

The posterior facets can be seen on X-ray but only to a limited extent. Degenerative changes and hypertrophy of the facets can be visualized to a greater extent on CT and MRI. Radio-opaque dye can also be injected into the joint and the distribution of the dye measured.

Figure 2.3 Transverse view of L2 showing normal intervertebral disc morphology

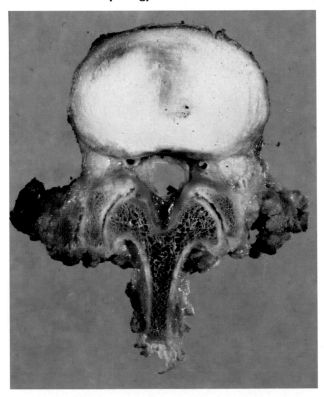

This section illustrates the central nucleus pulposus and outer annulus of the disc. The posterior facets are visible. The central canal is smaller than usual for this vertebral level. Courtesy Churchill-Livingstone (Saunders) Press

Figure 2.4 Longitudinal view of the lumbar spine showing normal disc size and morphology

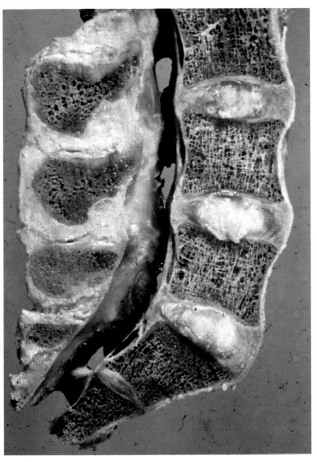

Courtesy Churchill-Livingstone (Saunders) Press

Figure 2.5 Normal discogram

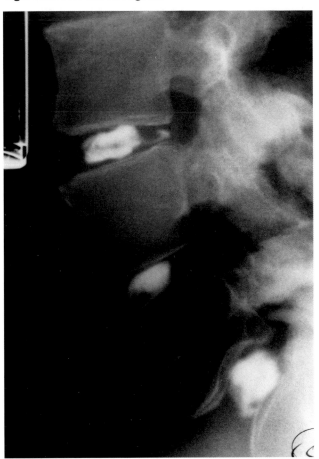

Lateral view following three-level discography. None of the discs were painful during injection. There is normal contrast dispersal in the nuclear compartment at each level

Figure 2.6 Normal discogram

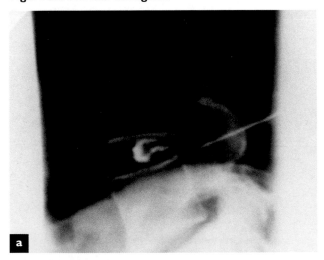

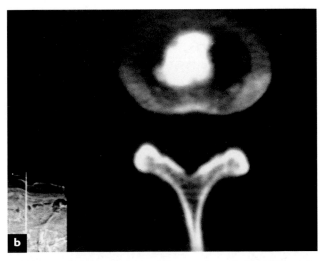

(a) Lateral radiograph with needle placement in the L4–L5 disc space following contrast injection; (b) post-discography CT scan in the same patient demonstrating normal contrast dispersal pattern in the nucleus

THE SPINAL LIGAMENTS AND MUSCLES

The vertebrae are connected by a series of longitudinally oriented ligaments. The most important ligament from a clinical perspective is the posterior longitudinal ligament, which connects to the vertebral bodies and posterior aspect of the vertebral disc and forms the anterior wall of the spinal canal. The ligamentum flavum, which has a higher elastin content, attaches between the lamina of the vertebra and extends into the anterior capsule of the zygapophyseal joints; it attaches to the pedicles above and below, forming the posterior wall of the vertebral canal and part of the roof of the lateral foramina through which the nerve roots pass. There are also dense fibrous ligaments connecting the spinous processes and the transverse processes, as well as a number of ligaments attaching the lower lumbar vertebrae to the sacrum and pelvis.

The musculature of the spine is similar in microscopic structures to that of other skeletal muscles. The individual muscle cells have small peripherally located nuclei and are filled with the contractile proteins, actin and myosin. The actin and myosin form cross-striations, which are easily visualized on light microscopy of longitudinal sections of muscle. The sarcomeres formed by the actin and myosin fibrils are separated by Z-lines, to which the actin is attached, and are visible on electron microscopy. The nuclei of the muscle cells are thin, elongated and arranged along the periphery of the cells.

The muscles of the back are arranged in three layers. The most superficial, or *outer layer*, is made up of large fleshy erector spinae muscles, which attach to the iliac and sacral crests inferiorly and to the spinous processes throughout the spine. In the lower lumbar region, it is a single muscle, but it divides into three distinct columns of muscles, separated by fibrous tissue. Below the erector spinae muscles is an *intermediate muscle group*, made up of three layers that collectively form the multifidus muscle. These muscles originate from the sacrum and the mamillary processes that expand backwards from the lumbar pedicles. They extend cranially and medially to insert into the lamina and adjacent spinous processes, one, two or three levels above their origin. The *deep muscular layer* consists of small muscles arranged from one level to another between the spinous processes, transverse processes and mamillary processes and the lamina. In the lumbar spine, there are also large anterior and lateral muscles including the quadratus lumborum, psoas and iliacus muscles which attach to the anterior vertebral bodies and transverse processes.

THE NERVE ROOTS AND SPINAL CORD

The spinal canal contains and protects the spinal cord and the spinal nerves. The spinal cord projects distally through the spinal canal from the brain, to taper out at the lower first or upper second lumbar vertebral level. The lower level of the spinal cord is known as the conus medullaris, from which nerve roots descend through the spinal canal to their respective exit points. The spinal cord is ensheathed

Figure 2.7 Transverse section of normal skeletal muscle

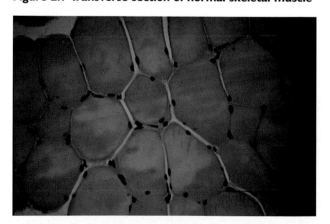

Light microscopy. Note the small peripheral nuclei situated at the periphery of the muscle cells Courtesy Churchill-Livingstone (Saunders) Press

Figure 2.8 Longitudinal section of normal skeletal muscle

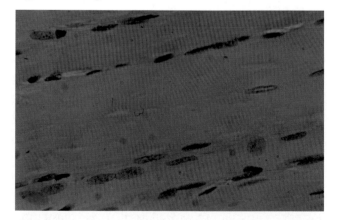

Light microscopy. Note the cross-striations and thin dark nuclei arranged along the periphery of the muscle cells. Courtesy Churchill-Livingstone (Saunders) Press

Figure 2.9 Diagram of sarcomere morphology

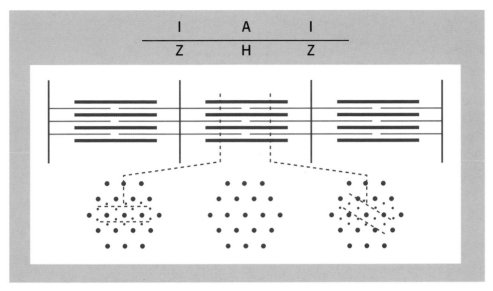

Note the location of the Z-lines and the interaction between the thin actin filaments and the thicker myosin filaments. Courtesy Churchill-Livingstone (Saunders) Press

by the three layers of the meninges. The pia mater invests the conus medullaris and rootlets. The outer layer, or dura mater, is separated by a potential subdural space to the arachnoid meninges. The subarachnoid space, which separates it from the pia mater, is filled with cerebrospinal fluid, which circulates up and down the spinal canal. The dura mater and pia mater continue distally, ensheathing the spinal nerves to the exit points. The spinal nerves exit the spinal cord by two nerve roots. The ventral nerve root carries motor fibers which originate in the anterior horn of the spinal cord. These neurons receive direct input from motor centers in the brain and, in turn, innervate the body musculature. The sensory or dorsal nerve root carries impulses from sensory receptors in the skin, muscles and other tissues of the body to the spinal cord and from there to the brain. The cell bodies of these sensory neurons are located within the dorsal root ganglia, which can be seen as an expansion within the dorsal root. The ventral and dorsal roots join to form the spinal nerve which exits the spinal canal and immediately divides into an anterior and posterior primary division. The posterior primary division, or ramus, of the nerve root innervates the facet joints and the posterior musculature, as well as the major posterior ligaments. The anterior primary division, or ramus, gives rise to nerves that innervate the intervertebral disc and the anterior longitudinal ligaments, and

Figure 2.10 Normal muscle morphology

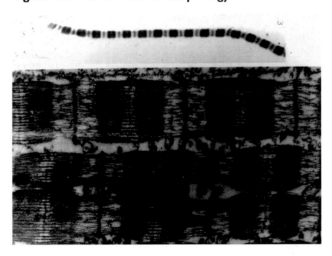

Electron microscopy of muscle, longitudinal section, showing dark vertical Z-lines separated by lighter actin and darker myosin filaments to make up the sarcomere. Courtesy Churchill-Livingstone (Saunders) Press

sends nerve fibers via the gray ramus communicans to the sympathetic ganglion chain. A small sinuvertebral, or recurrent nerve of Von Luschka, branches from the mixed spinal nerve to innervate the posterior longitudinal ligament. The anterior primary division then travels laterally or inferiorly, depending on the vertebral level, to form the various plexuses and nerves that innervate muscles

Figure 2.11 Normal muscle morphology showing mitochondria

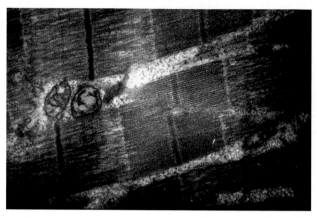

Longitudinal section electron microscopy showing three normal muscle fibers from a cat. The Z-lines and muscle filaments are evident. Mitochondria can be seen in the septa between the muscle fibers. Courtesy Churchill-Livingstone (Saunders) Press

Figure 2.12 Normal muscle anatomy, thecal sac and dorsal root ganglion

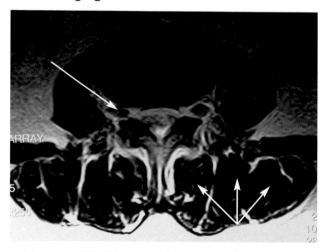

Axial lumbar MR T2 weighted image at L4–L5 disc space demonstrating a normal-appearing thecal sac. The dorsal root ganglion of the exiting L5 nerve root is seen (arrow). The posterior paraspinal muscles are seen: multifidus, longissimus thoracis pars lumborum, and iliocostalis lumborum pars lumborum (arrows). The psoas muscle is demonstrated at the anterolateral aspect of the vertebra

throughout the body. Inflammatory processes occurring within the disc activate nociceptive nerve endings which send impulses via the sinu-vertebral nerve and gray ramus communicans nerve to the spinal cord. Inflammatory changes occurring in the facet joints or dorsal muscles and ligaments activate

Figure 2.13 Normal thecal sac, S1 nerve root and sacroiliac joint

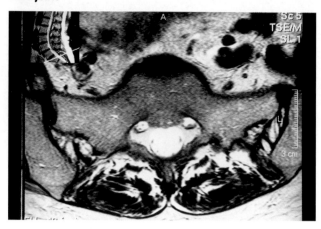

Sagittal MRI at the level of the upper border of the sacrum demonstrating normal posterior paraspinal muscle compartment, sacroiliac joint and thecal sac

Figure 2.14 Paraspinal and posterior musculature

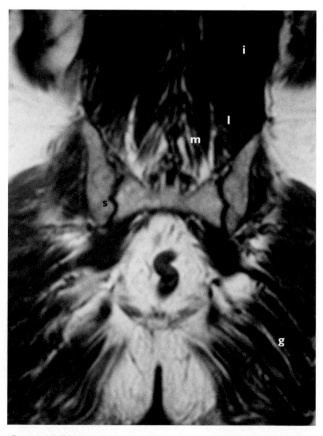

Coronal MRI reveals details of the posterior paraspinal muscles and their insertion onto the upper border of the sacrum and posterior ilium. The multifidus (m), longissimus thoracis pars lumborum (l), and iliocostalis (i), and gluteus maximum (g) are seen. The sacroiliac joints are visible (s)

Figure 2.15 Normal-appearing intrathecal rootlets and basivertebral vein channels

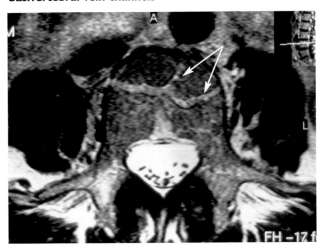

Axial T2 weighed MR image at the pedicle level of L4. The rootlets of the cauda equina are seen in the posterior thecal sac, with the sacral rootlets more posterior in position, and the L5 rootlets positioned laterally. The basivertebral vein complex entry into the L4 vertebra (arrows) and the venous channels are visible

nociceptive fibers which travel within the dorsal primary division of the spinal nerve.

Injury or entrapment of the neural elements of the spine can result in loss of function of a single motor or sensory nerve root, if the entrapment is within the neural foramen. If the entrapment is due to stenosis or narrowing of the central canal, function within the cauda equina or spinal cord can be affected. Injury to the spinal cord can impact on the reflex centers or the sensory and motor pathways to the central control centers in the brain.

The central canal of the spine can be well visualized and measured on either CT or MRI scan. The spinal cord and the nerve roots in the cauda equina can also be visualized using these imaging techniques. The nerve roots, as they exit through the foramen, can be best seen on MRI scan and the size of the nerve root canal, which has the potential to entrap these nerves, can be measured. There is, however, marked variation in the size of the central canal and lateral foramina through which the spinal cord and nerve roots pass. The simple measurement

Figure 2.16 The innervation of the anterior spinal structures

Nucleus pulposus

Anterior longitudinal ligament

Sympathetic ganglion

Gray ramus communicans

Annulus fibrosis

Sinu-vertebral nerve

Spinal nerve

Anterior primary division

Posterior longitudinal ligament

Posterior primary division

Dura mater

Dorsal root ganglion

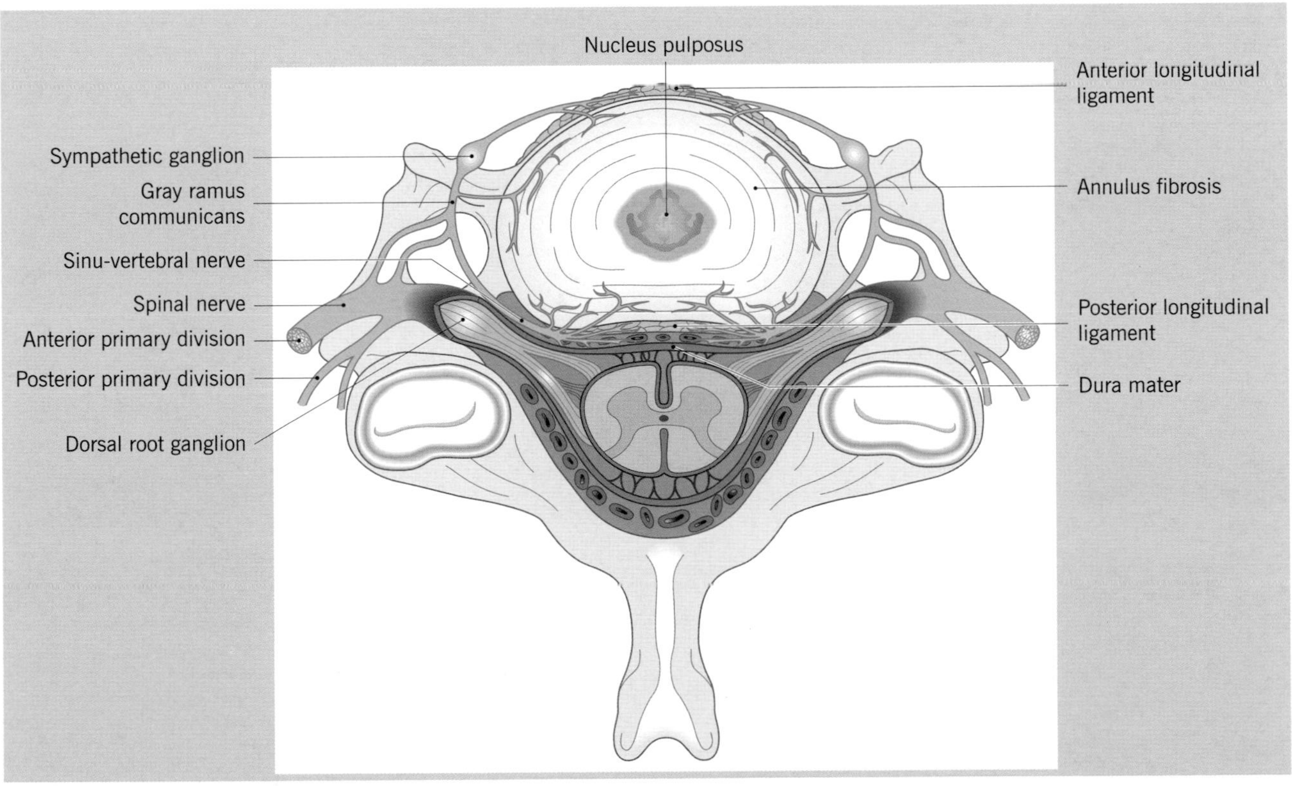

The nerve root separates into an anterior and posterior primary division. The anterior spinal structures receive their innervation from branches originating from the anterior primary division via the recurrent sinu-vertebral nerve and the gray ramus communicans

Figure 2.17 The innervation of the posterior spinal structures

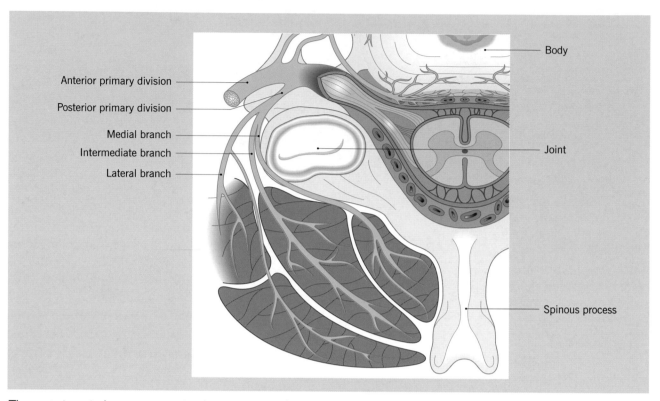

The posterior spinal structures receive their innervation from the medial, intermediate and lateral branches of the posterior primary division of the nerve root

Figure 2.18 Lateral view of the innervation of the spine

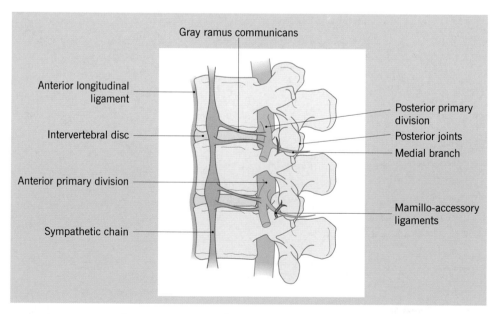

The gray ramus communicans connects the primary anterior division of the nerve root with the sympathetic chain. The medial branch of the posterior primary division passes under a small mamillo-accessory ligament before innervating the medial spinal muscles

Figure 2.19 The innervation of the pelvic structures by the lower sacral and pudendal nerves

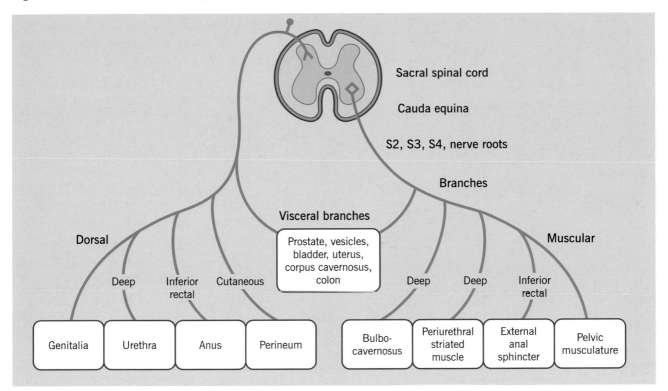

The S2, S3 and S4 spinal nerves travel through the cauda equina from the sacral spinal cord to provide motor, sensory and autonomic innervation to the pelvic and genital structures

Figure 2.20 The recording of H-reflexes

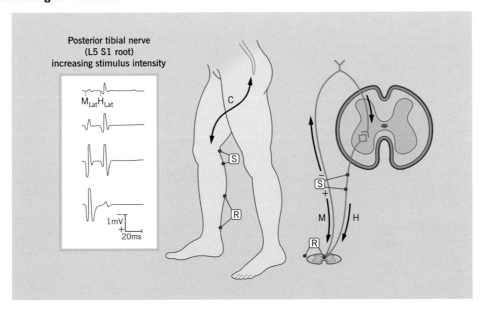

S1 nerve root function can be assessed by measuring the H-reflex from the soleus/gastrocnemius muscle on stimulation of the posterior tibial nerve at the popliteal fossa. The latency represents the time it takes for nerve impulses to travel from the point of stimulation to the spinal cord. Entrapment or injury to the S1 nerve root or sciatic nerve will either decrease the amplitude and/or prolong the latency of the response

Figure 2.21 The recording of F-responses

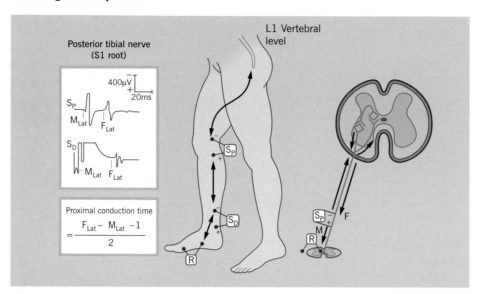

Proximal nerve function that includes the nerve root can be assessed by measuring the F-response from distal muscles innervated by a mixed or primary motor nerve. The nerve impulses travel through the spinal cord and connect with a Renshaw interneuron to send impulses back along the motor nerve to the distal muscles. The proximal conduction time represents the time it takes for nerve impulses to travel from the point of stimulation to the spinal cord and back to the point of stimulation. Any entrapment or injury to the nerve root or sciatic nerve will prolong the latency of the response

Figure 2.22 The complexity of the sciatic nerve

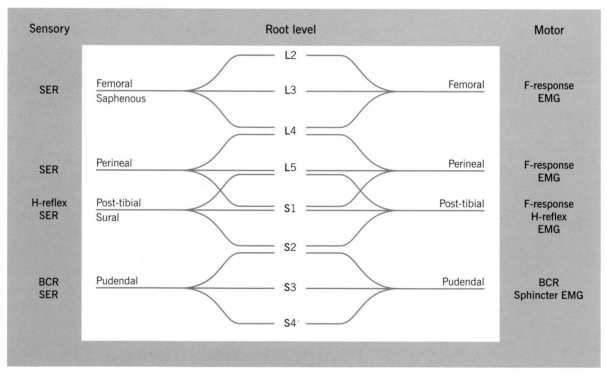

This diagram illustrates the difficulty in isolating an injury or entrapment of a single nerve root using a single electrodiagnostic test. The peripheral nerves receive input from multiple nerve roots. Electrodiagnostic testing often requires a battery of tests, as noted

Figure 2.23 Somatosensory evoked responses

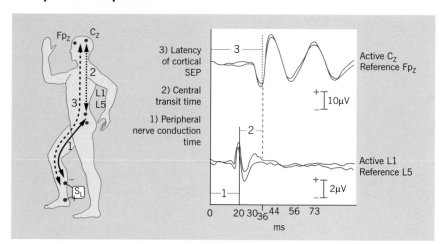

Cortical somatosensory evoked potentials (SEP) can be measured over the scalp using surface electrodes and computer averaging on stimulation of most peripheral sensory nerves. This diagram illustrates the response on stimulation of the posterior tibial nerve at the ankle. It is often possible to record a response over the lumbar spine as well as the scalp. The difference in latency between the spinal response and the cortical response is known as the central conduction time (CCT), and represents the time that an impulse requires to travel from the spinal cord to the brain

Figure 2.24 The four divisions of the nervous system that control bowel, bladder and sexual function

Central sensory
Cortical evoked responses
Electroencephalography

Central motor
Cystometry
Colonometry
Noctural penile tumescence

Peripheral sensory
Sensory conduction
Spinal evoked responses
Cystometry
Bulbocavernosus reflex

Peripheral motor
Bulbocavernosus reflex
Cystometry
Colonometry
Sphincter EMG

The clinical physiological tests that can be used to assess the integrity of these pathways are listed

of the size of the canals does not confirm the presence or absence of dysfunction within the spinal cord or nerve root. In order to achieve this, it is necessary to conduct a clinical examination and, where necessary, electrodiagnostic studies.

The diagnostic field known as clinical neurophysiology encompasses a series of testing procedures used to detect and quantify nerve function. The primary electrodiagnostic study utilized to document nerve root entrapment or injury is electromyography, where a needle is inserted into the muscle and the presence of denervation of the muscle can be documented. Nerve root compression results in irritability of the cell membranes of a muscle. This can be noted on electromyography as short fibrillation potentials and positive sharp waves, which are not seen in normally innervated muscles. Within a few months following denervation, the remaining intact nerves begin to sprout collateral nerve fibers to innervate those muscles that have lost their nerve supply. This process results in a change in the appearance of the normal muscle activity seen on electromyography, which takes on a polyphasic appearance. S1 nerve root function can also be determined by measuring neural reflexes, which travel to the spinal cord on stimulation of the sciatic nerve in the popliteal fossa, and by recording the motor response generated from these H-reflexes in the gastrocnemius muscles. The F-response is another method of measuring the motor pathway in the nerve roots which travels from a point of stimulation over a peripheral nerve to the spinal cord and back to the muscle. A battery of these tests is often necessary to localize the nerve root that is affected, because peripheral nerves and muscles are often innervated by multiple nerve roots which join within the sciatic and brachial plexuses. The documentation of nerve pathways within the spinal cord is achieved by stimulating a peripheral sensory nerve and recording electrical responses, using computer averaging over the spine and over the brain. Delay or absence of these somatosensory evoked responses or potentials is strongly suggestive of a lesion impacting on the sensory pathways within the spinal cord. The differentiation of peripheral nerve lesions or injury distal to the nerve root is achieved by measuring nerve conduction in peripheral nerves. The documentation of nerve injury or entrapment, affecting bowel, bladder and/or sexual function and numbness in the perineum and genitalia, can be made by stimulating the pudendal nerve and recording the bulbocavernosis reflex and cortical evoked potentials. Direct measurement of bladder function using cystometry, bowel function using colonometry and male sexual function using nocturnal penile tumescence and rigidity may also be of value if it is suspected that these functions are being affected by lesions in the cauda equina or spinal cord.

BIBLIOGRAPHY

Bogduk N. The innervation of the lumbar spine. *Spine* 1983;8:286

Bogduk N, Twomey LT. *Clinical Anatomy of the Lumbar Spine*, 2nd edn. New York: Churchill Livingstone, 1991

Haldeman S, Dvorak J. Clinical neurophysiology and electrodiagnostic testing in low back pain. *The Lumbar Spine*, Vol 1, 2nd edn. The International Society for the Study of the Lumbar Spine Editorial Committee. Philadelphia: WB Saunders Co, 1996

3

Spinal degeneration

Degenerative changes within the spine are the most common pathological finding noted on autopsy and on imaging of the spine. The process of degenerative change occurs in the entire population as it ages and is probably part of the normal aging process. The speed and extent of the degenerative changes appear to be impacted by hereditary factors as well as specific and continuous traumatic events that occur through a person's life. Even the most severe degenerative changes can occur in the absence of symptomatology, but back pain is more common in individuals who demonstrate these degenerative changes. It appears that the degenerative changes in the spine make one more vulnerable to the inflammatory effects of trauma.

Degenerative changes are most evident in the intervertebral discs and the facet joints, usually at the same time, but often to varying degrees. It is useful to visualize the vertebral motion-segment as a 'three-joint complex' in which degenerative changes in the posterior facets impact the intervertebral disc, and pathological changes within the intervertebral disc will create greater stressors upon the posterior facet joints.

THE INTERVERTEBRAL DISC

Degenerative changes within the intervertebral disc usually start as small circumferential tears in the annulus fibrosus. These annular tears increase in size and coalesce to form radial fissures. The radial fissures then expand and extend into the nucleus pulposus, disrupting the disc structure internally. There is a loss of proteoglycans and water content from the nucleus which results in a loss of the height

Figure 3.1 Early stage of disc degeneration, high signal intensity zone

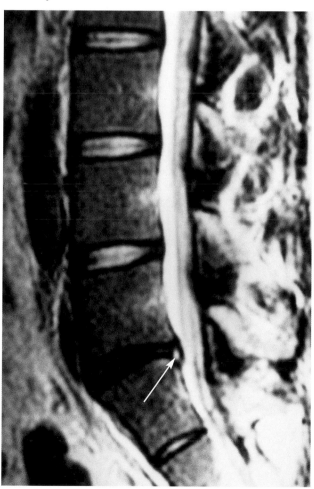

Sagittal T2 weighed MR image of lumbar spine demonstrating a normal-appearing signal of all discs except the L5 disc where there is a high signal intensity zone in the posterior aspect of the disc space (arrow). This represents nuclear material that has extended through a confluence of annular tears, leading to a radial fissure in the disc

Figure 3.2 Stage-one degeneration of the lumbar three-joint complex

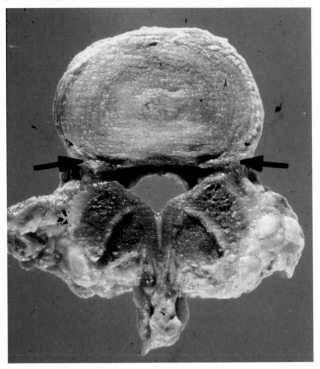

There are two small circumferential tears in the posterior annulus (arrows). This represents stage one of the degenerative process in the discs. The posterior facets are enlarged and the facets show degenerative changes. This demonstrates the interaction between the discs and the posterior joints. Courtesy Churchill-Livingstone (Saunders) Press

of the disc. As degeneration continues, the disc collapses, shortening the distance between the two vertebral bodies. This re-absorption can progress to the point where the vertebral bodies are eventually separated only by dense sclerotic fibrous tissue which is all that remains of the original disc structure.

At the same time as the disc is being reabsorbed, the vertebral bodies on either side of the disc become dense and sclerotic. Osteophytes extend from the vertebral bodies around its circumference, presumably in an attempt to stabilize the three-joint complex and reduce motion. Occasionally, the osteophytes may join and fuse, resulting in bony ankylosis of the joint.

THE FACET JOINTS

Degenerative changes within the posterior facet usually begin with an inflammatory synovitis, which

Figure 3.3 Stage-two degeneration of the three-joint complex

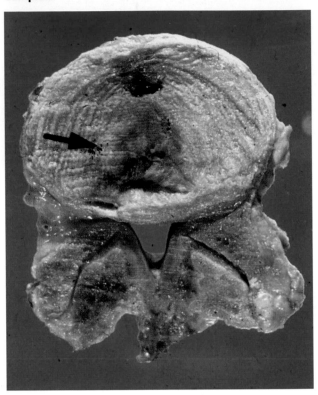

This cross-section of the lumbar spine shows degenerative changes in the intervertebral disc and the posterior facet joints. The extensive degenerative changes in the posterior joints have resulted in enlargement of the facets. On the left side of the disc near the back of the vertebral body, there is a small circumferential tear in the annulus fibrosus. This tear has enlarged and spread to the center of the disc. Courtesy Churchill-Livingstone (Saunders) Press

can lead to the formation of a synovial fold, projecting into the joint between the cartilage surfaces. There is gradual thinning of the cartilage, which starts in the periphery with progressive loss of cartilage tissue. Subperiosteal osteophytes begin to form which enlarge both the inferior and superior facets. This breakdown continues until there is almost total loss of articular cartilage with marked periarticular fibrosis and the formation of subperiosteal new bone expanding the volume of the superior and inferior facets. During the early phases of these degenerative changes, the facet capsule can become very lax, allowing increased movement. It is probably this period of increased mobility of the joint which leads to further degeneration within the posterior facets, and puts further stress on the intervertebral discs.

Figure 3.4 Stage-three degeneration of the lumbar intervertebral disc

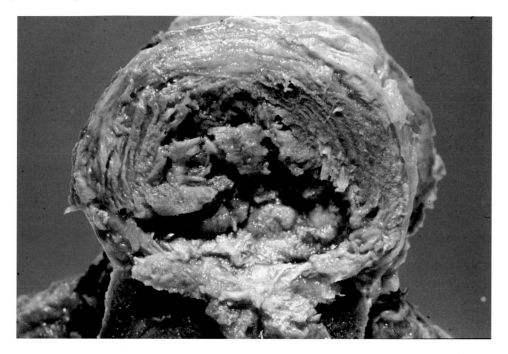

This cross-section through a lumbar disc shows very marked degenerative changes. There is complete disintegration of the nucleus pulposus. These changes have resulted in instability of the three-joint complex at this level. Courtesy Churchill-Livingstone (Saunders) Press

Figure 3.5 Complete disintegration of the lumbar intervertebral disc

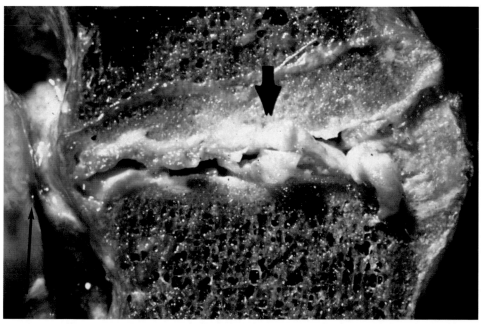

This longitudinal section of a lumbar disc at L4–L5 shows marked degeneration, with almost complete disintegration of the disc (short arrow). The lumbar spine is markedly unstable at this level. The thickened annulus fibrosus is bulging around the circumference of the disc with resultant stenosis and narrowing of the spinal canal (long arrow). Courtesy Churchill-Livingstone (Saunders) Press

Figure 3.6 Intervertebral disc resorption

Figure 3.7 Multilevel disc disruption

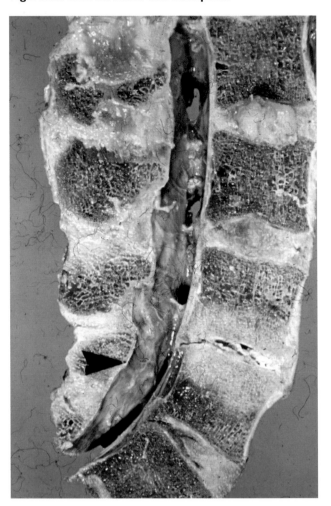

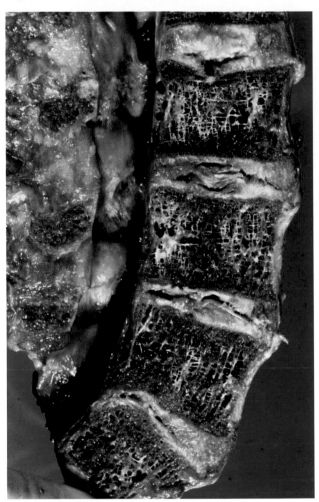

Longitudinal section through the lumbar spine at L4–L5. There is almost complete resorption of the disc which is seen as a small slit between the vertebral bodies. There is sclerosis of the bone in the vertebral bodies on either side of the disc. Courtesy Churchill-Livingstone (Saunders) Press

Longitudinal sagittal section of the lumbar spine showing marked degeneration at four levels. There is a Schmorl's node at the upper level at L2–L3, with herniation of the nucleus pulposus into the vertebral body. There is disintegration of the L3–L4 and L4–L5 discs. At the L5–S1 level, there is disc resorption, with sclerotic bone on either side of the remnants of the disc. Courtesy Churchill-Livingstone (Saunders) Press

IMAGING OF DEGENERATIVE CHANGES

Degenerative change in the intervertebral disc is best visualized in its early stages on MRI scan. T2 weighted MR images of the lumbar spine measure the hydration status of the disc, which gradually decreases in the presence of degenerative changes. This results in a change in the signal intensity within the disc, which is easily seen. Radial and circumferential tears can also be visualized on MR images. On CT scan imaging, gas formation can be seen within the radial tears and the annulus during the reabsorption phase.

As degenerative changes progress, narrowing of the disc space from disc reabsorption can be noted on standard X-rays, as can the growth of circumferential osteophytes. Sclerotic changes within the facet joints can also be noted on standard X-rays. Better visualization of these changes is achieved by means of CT scan or MR images, which can document the growth of osteophytic spurs and determine whether they encroach on the spinal canal or neuroforamina.

Figure 3.8 Degenerative posterior (apophyseal) joint

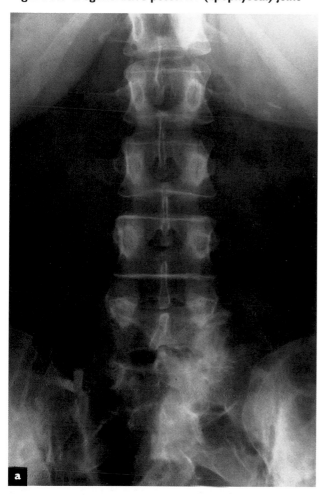

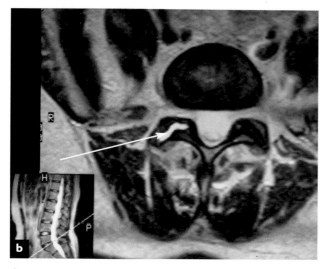

Anteroposterior view of the lumbar spine demonstrating increased radiodensity in the right L5–S1 posterior facet (apophyseal) joint (a). On the axial T2 magnetic resonance image, there is increased signal intensity in the right posterior (apophyseal) joint, consistent with increased synovial fluid (arrow) (b)

Figure 3.9 Degenerative spondylosis on CT scan

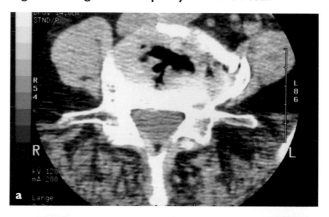

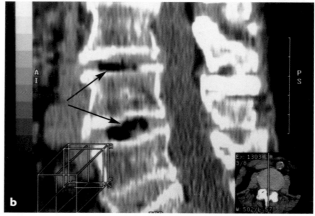

Axial (a) and sagittal (b) computed tomography images of degenerative lumbar spondylosis. The intervertebral disc has lost height, and there is gas in the disc space which appears black on CT images (arrow). On the axial image, there is lateral protrusion of the disc margin to the left

Figure 3.10 Degenerative disc disease

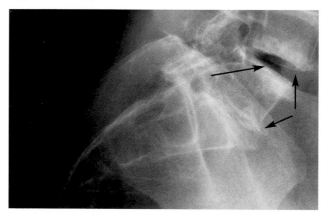

Lateral radiograph of lumbar spine demonstrating increased radiodensity across the endplates of the L4–L5 and L5–S1 vertebrae. The Knuttson gas phenomenon is present at L4–L5 (arrow), indicative of advanced degeneration of the L4–L5 disc. There are traction spurs anteriorly at L4–L5 (arrows) and L5–S1, which occur with segmental instability

Figure 3.11 Early degenerative changes in the posterior joint

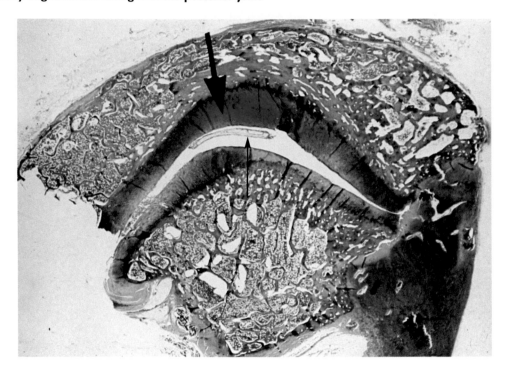

This light microscopic cross-sectional view through the facet joint shows very early degenerative changes in the posterior joint. The purple-staining articular cartilage represents normal cartilage. The arrow points to a thin sausage-shaped tag of synovial tissue lying between the articular surfaces. Courtesy Churchill-Livingstone (Saunders) Press

Figure 3.12 Intermediate degeneration of the posterior joint

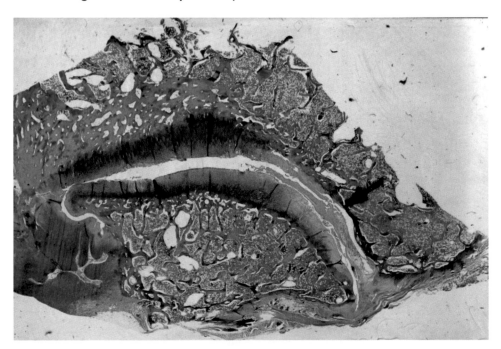

Light microscopic cross-section of the posterior facet joint. The arrow points to thin degenerate cartilage on the upper part of the joint. A large thick fibrofatty tag extends from the joint capsule on the right, lying between the two purple articular surfaces. Courtesy Churchill-Livingstone (Saunders) Press

Figure 3.13 Advanced degeneration of the posterior joint

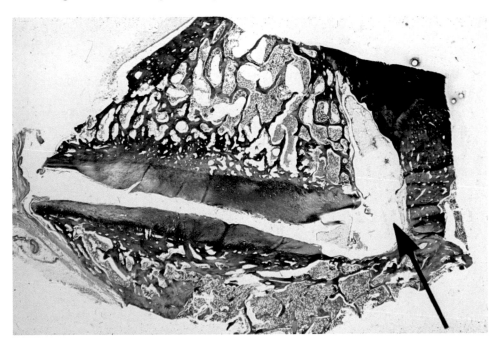

Light microscopic view of the posterior facet joint showing advanced degenerative changes. There is thinning of the articular cartilage on the lower joint surface, with a large space between the joint capsule and the articular surfaces. This is indicative of a lax capsule and an unstable joint. Courtesy Churchill-Livingstone (Saunders) Press

Figure 3.14 Degeneration and fusion of the posterior joint

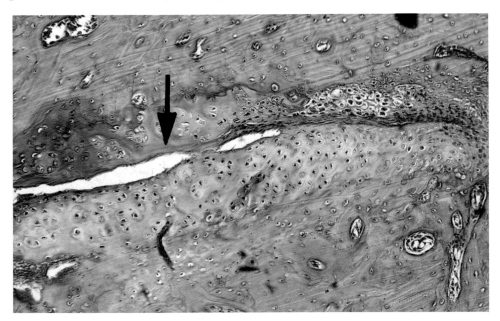

Light microscopic section through the posterior joint showing marked degeneration. The joint is almost obliterated and there is cartilagineous fusion of the two facets of the joint. The arrow points to the remnants of the joint space. This type of change occurs when there has been immobilization of the joint for prolonged periods. Courtesy Churchill-Livingstone (Saunders) Press

Figure 3.15 Degeneration and subluxation of the posterior joint

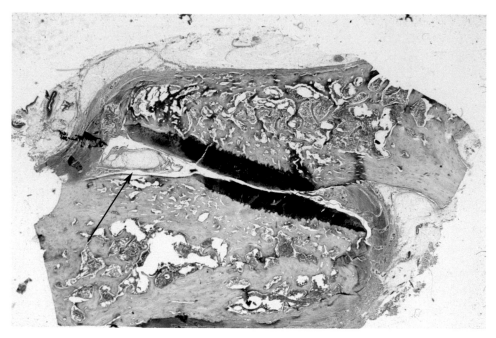

Light microscopic cross-sectional view of a degenerated posterior joint. The two surfaces of the articular cartilage have slid past each other, resulting in subluxation of the joint. On the left side, a fibrofatty tag of synovium attached to the joint capsule extends into the joint (arrow). Courtesy Churchill-Livingstone (Saunders) Press

Figure 3.16 Degeneration with hypertrophy of the posterior joint

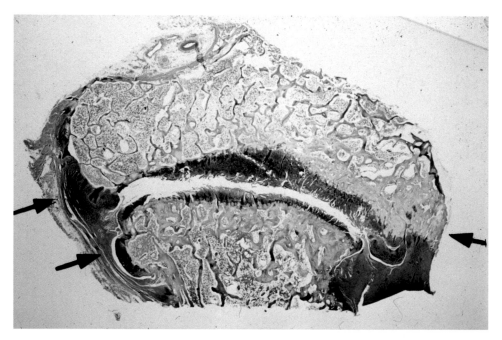

Light microscopic cross-sectional view of a posterior joint showing extensive hypertrophy and enlargement of the bones of the facets. The purple articular cartilage on both sides of the joint is very thin and fragmented. The arrows point to the grossly thickened capsule on both sides of the joint. Courtesy Churchill-Livingstone (Saunders) Press

Figure 3.17 Degeneration causing foraminal encroachment

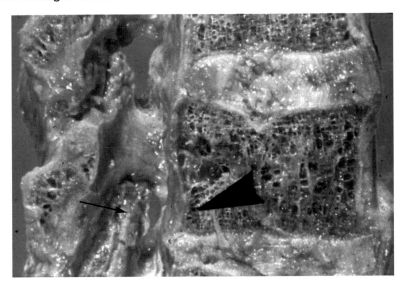

Longitudinal sagittal section through the lumbar spine at the L4–L5 level showing advanced degeneration of the intervertebral disc and the posterior facets. The intervertebral foramen (large arrow) is much reduced in size as the result of impingement by an enlarged superior articular process of the facet of L5 (small arrow). Courtesy Churchill Livingstone (Saunders) Press

Figure 3.18 Degeneration of the disc and posterior joints causing foraminal narrowing

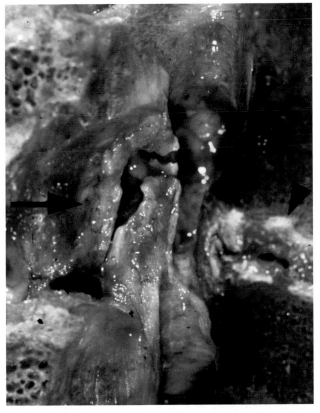

Longitudinal sagittal view of the lumbar spine at the L4–L5 level showing marked degenerative changes in the posterior facet joint and the intervertebral disc. There is entrapment of the synovium within the joint (left arrow). The breakdown in the disc is evident (right arrow) with bulging posteriorly. The spinal canal is narrowed due to the combined effects of the joint hypertrophy and the bulging disc. Courtesy Churchill-Livingstone (Saunders) Press

Figure 3.19 Facet joint cyst

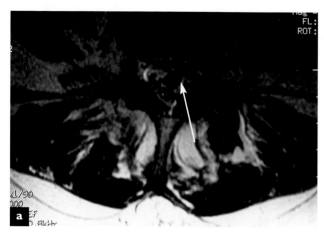

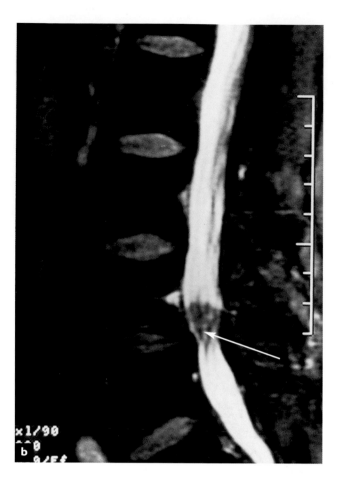

Axial (a) and sagittal (b) T2 weighted MR images of a facet joint cyst originating from the left L4–L5 facet joint (arrow) causing significant mass effect against the thecal sac

BIBLIOGRAPHY

Alam F, Moss SG, Schweitzer ME. Imaging of degenerative disease of the lumbar spine and related conditions. *Semin Spine Surg* 1999;11:76

Bernard TN. Using computed tomography and enhanced magnetic resonance imaging to distinguish between scar tissue and recurrent lumbar disc herniation. *Spine* 1994;19:2826

Kirkaldy-Willis WH, Wedge JH, Yong-Hing K, Reilly J. Pathology and pathogenesis of lumbar spondylosis. *Spine* 1978;3:319

Modic MT, Steinberg PM, Ross JS, Masaryk TJ, Carter JR. Degenerative disk disease: assessment of changes in vertebral body marrow with MR imaging. *Radiology* 1988;166:193

Osti OL, Vernon-Roberts B, Moore R, Fraser RD. Annular tears and disc degeneration in the lumbar spine. *J Bone Joint Surg* 1992;74-B:678

Selby DK, Paris SV. Anatomy of facet joints and its clinical correlation with low back pain. *Contemp Orthop* 1981;3:1097

4

Acute trauma

Acute trauma, either in the form of a direct blow to the spine or the application of excessive rotational or compressive force applied to the spine, can result in injury to virtually any structure. The structures most vulnerable to acute trauma are the annulus fibrosus of the intervertebral discs, the endplates of the intervertebral discs and the vertebral bodies.

DISC HERNIATION

When compressive or rotational forces are applied to the spine, the fibers of the annulus fibrosus can be stretched beyond their elastic capacity and tear. If these tears are oriented in a radial fashion, the nucleus pulposus may migrate through the tear, causing a protrusion of the disc beyond its natural borders. This can occur as an acute process in a healthy disc given sufficient force. Degenerated discs that already have some degree of annular tearing, usually in a circumferential pattern, have less elastic proteoglycans and are less able to withstand these forces. If there is a disruption of the posterior longitudinal ligament, nuclear material can extrude through the annulus, narrowing the diameter of the

Figure 4.1 Central disc herniation

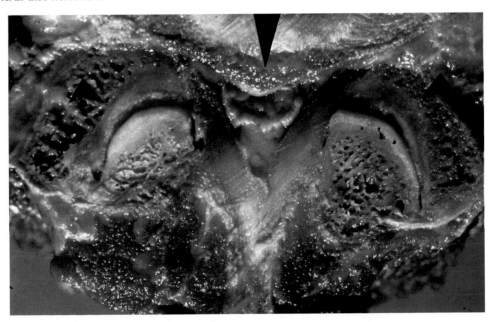

Transverse section at the L5–S1 level showing a disc herniation centrally encroaching on the central canal, causing stenosis. Courtesy Churchill-Livingstone (Saunders) Press

Figure 4.2 Schmorl's node

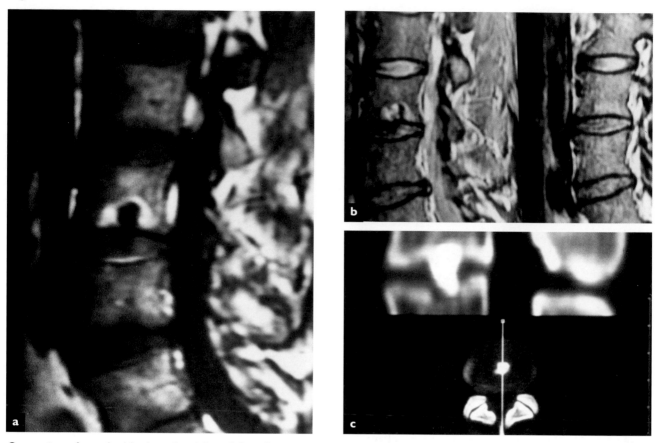

One variety of vertebral body and endplate defect allowing herniation of the nucleus pulposus into the vertebral body. (a) MRI T1 weighted image revealed herniation of the L3–L4 disc into the L3 body, creating a 'Schmorl's node' or 'Geipel hernia'; (b) the same patient's T2 weighed image; (c) post-discogram computed tomography sagittal reformation demonstrating a 'Schmorl's node'

Figure 4.3 Herniated nucleus pulposus L5–S1

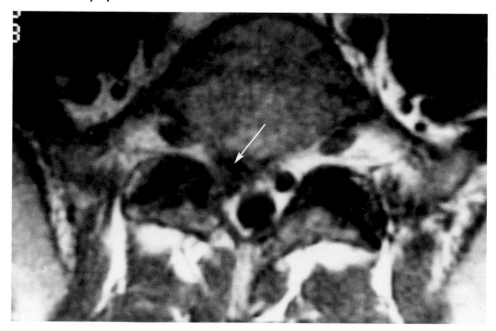

Axial MRI demonstrating a right-sided herniated nucleus pulposus displacing the S1 nerve root (arrow)

Figure 4.4 Lateral lumbar disc herniation

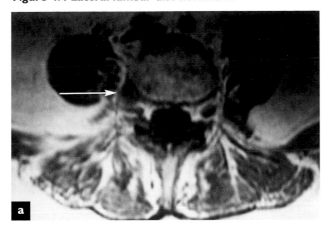

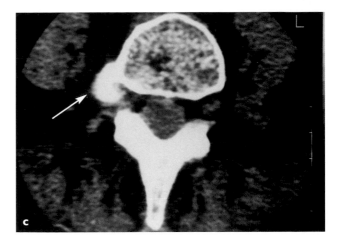

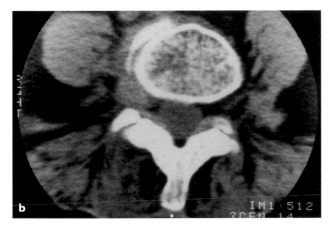

Demonstration of three different imaging techniques. (a) MRI demonstrates a right-sided lateral disc herniation. The disc protrusion effaces the dorsal root ganglion (arrow); (b) non-enhanced computed tomography of the same patient reveals increased signal density of the lateral disc herniation; (c) post-discography computed tomography of the same patient demonstrates contrast enhancement of the lateral disc herniation (arrow)

Figure 4.5 Large extruded midline disc herniation

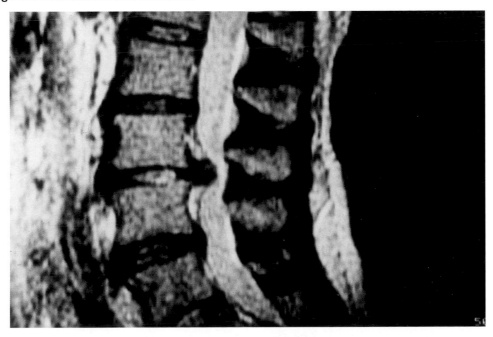

MRI demonstrates a central disc extrusion at L3–L4. Note that the posterior longitudinal ligament has been elevated posteriorly and separated by the disc herniation. There is marked central canal stenosis caused by the disc herniation

Figure 4.6 Lateral disc herniation, normal nerve and muscle anatomy

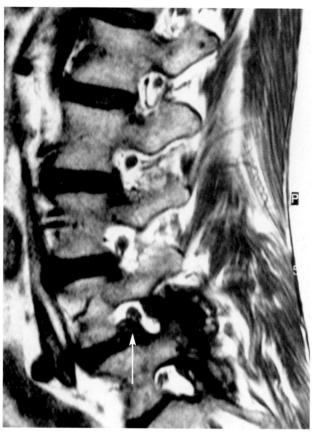

Sagittal T2 weighted MR image demonstrating a lateral disc herniation at L4–L5 displacing the exiting L4 nerve root (arrow). Note the relationship between the normal-appearing nerve roots at L2 and L3 and the pedicle. The attachment of the longissimus thoracic pars lumborum to the transverse process is seen in the posterior paraspinal muscle compartment

Figure 4.8 Radial fissure

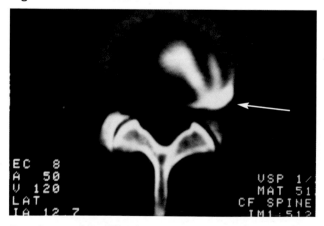

Post-discography CT demonstrating contrast extending through a confluence of annular tears into a radial fissure, with outer annular contrast enhancement (arrow)

Figure 4.7 Lumbar disc herniation

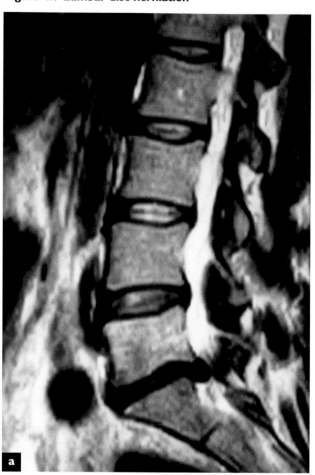

a

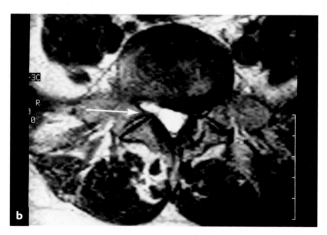

b

Sagittal T2 weighted MR image of a lumbar disc herniation at L5–SI (a). Axial MR image demonstrating the L5–SI disc herniation to the left, displacing the SI nerve root (b). The normal-appearing right SI nerve root is seen in the right subarticular recess (arrow)

Figure 4.9 Lumbar disc herniation

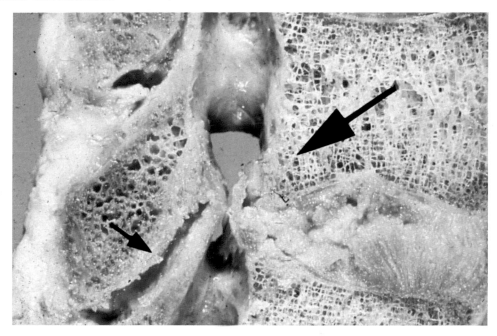

Longitudinal section through the lumbar spine showing a large disc herniation at L4–L5 (large arrow). The posterior facets show degenerative changes in the form of irregular surfaces (small arrow). Courtesy Churchill-Livingstone (Saunders) Press

Figure 4.10 Schmorl's node

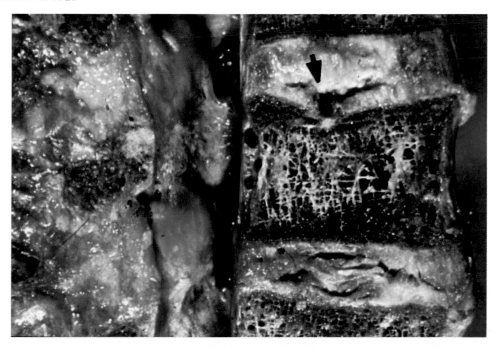

Longitudinal section through L2, L3, L4 showing degeneration and disruption of the intervertebral disc at these levels. The arrow points to a fracture in the endplate at the superior aspect of L3, resulting in herniation of the nucleus pulposus into the vertebral body

Figure 4.11 Compression fracture

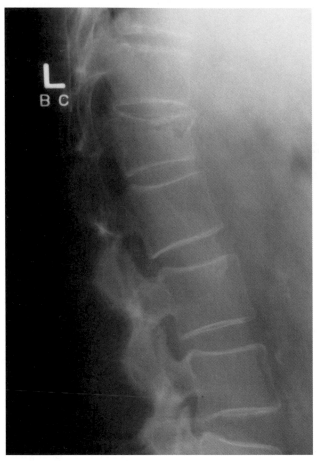

Lateral lumbar radiograph in a patient with osteoporosis and a compression fracture of L1, with collapse and wedging of the anterior aspect of the vertebral body

Figure 4.12 Compression fracture

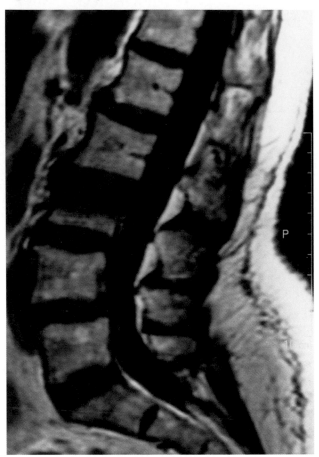

Sagittal T1 weighted MR demonstrating decreased signal intensity in the L3 vertebra, indicative of bone edema secondary to a compression fracture

neural canal. If the disc herniation protrudes posteriorly in the midline to narrow the central canal of the spine, compression of the cauda equina or spinal cord can occur. If the disc protrudes laterally, it can extend into the lateral foramina, encroaching on the nerve root.

COMPRESSION FRACTURE

A direct axial force applied to the spine, especially in flexion, can result in a collapse of the vertebral body. There is a disruption of the intrinsic bone structure, followed by edema and healing of the bone. If severe, these compression fractures can force spicules of bone or the entire vertebral body to move posteriorly, encroaching on the central canal or laterally encroaching on the neuroforamen.

As a result of compression forces, the endplate of the vertebral body may collapse, allowing herniation of the nucleus pulposus into the vertebral body. This has become known as a Schmorl's node.

Bony fractures of the vertebral body are well visualized on X-ray and the edema associated with healing is visible on MRI scan. Disc herniation, however, is not seen on standard X-ray and requires either an MRI or CT scan to be visualized. Radial tears and the protrusion of the nucleus into the tear can be visualized by injecting a radio-opaque dye into the disc, which can be visualized on X-ray as a discogram. These changes are more clearly seen on post-discography CT scanning.

Electrodiagnostic evaluation is often used to document injury or encroachment on the nerve roots or the spinal cord which occurs as a result of disc

Figure 4.13 Compression fracture

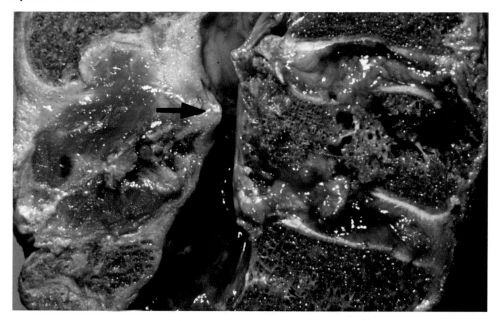

Longitudinal section from L4 to the sacrum. There is a compression fracture of L5 with posterior displacement of the fractured bone, leading to marked narrowing of the central canal (arrow). Courtesy Churchill-Livingstone (Saunders) Press

Figure 4.14 Abnormal electromyography potentials

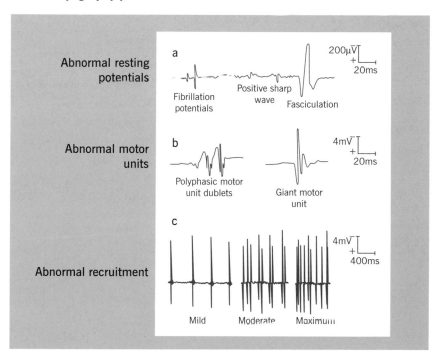

The upper line of potentials (a) represents the abnormalities following acute denervation of muscles. Muscles with intact nerve supply are normally silent at rest. The middle line of potentials (b) can be seen as a result of reinnervation of the nerve to the previously denervated muscle. These abnormal potentials may show multiple phases and/or large amplitude giant potentials and potentials that appear as duplets. The lower line of potentials (c) shows the response seen in a partially denervated muscle on voluntary contraction of the muscle. The number of potentials are markedly reduced compared to the normal interference pattern seen on normal muscle contraction

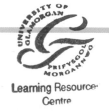

Learning Resource
Centre

Figure 4.15 Chronic electromyographic potentials

Left

Right

100   150   200
m/s

100   150   200
m/s

These EMG potentials were recorded from the gastrocnemius muscle in a patient with a chronic S1 radiculopathy in the left leg. The polyphasic potentials differ from the normal potentials recorded from the normal gastrocnemius muscle in the right leg

Figure 4.16 Cauda equina syndrome

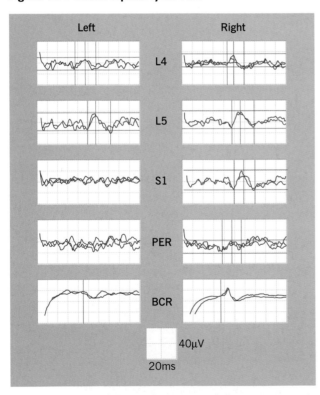

Left   Right

L4

L5

S1

PER

BCR

40µV

20ms

Electrodiagnostic studies from a patient with unilateral cauda equina injury secondary to a lumbar disc protrusion. The cortical somatosensory evoked potentials on stimulation of the S1 dermatome and the pudendal nerve are unobtainable on the symptomatic side, whereas the responses on stimulation of the L4 and L5 dermatomes are normal. There is also an abnormal bulbocavernosus reflex on the left or symptomatic side

herniation or fracture. Radiculopathy can be documented by noting denervation on needle electromyography of the muscles served by the involved nerve root. Nerve compression of the S1 nerve root can also result in a delay of the H-reflex on stimulation of the tibial nerve in the popliteal fossa. A delay in F-response can be noted in cauda equina syndrome or multiple level radiculopathy. Somatosensory evoked responses will show delayed or absence latency which can occur as a result of compression of the spinal cord or cauda equina.

BIBLIOGRAPHY

Spivak JM, Vaccaro AR, Cotler JM. Thoracolumbar spine trauma. I. Evaluation and classification. *J Am Acad Orthopaed Surg* 1995;3:345

Spivak JM, Vaccaro AR, Cotler JM. Thoracolumbar spine trauma. II. Principles of management. *J Am Acad Orthopaed Surg* 1995;3:353

Zamani MH, MacEwen GD. Herniation of the lumbar disc in children and adolescents. *J Pediatr Orthop* 1982;2:528

5

Chronic pathological changes

The effects of acute and cumulative trauma result in progressive degenerative changes that affect both the intervertebral disc and the posterior facets and can be found at multiple levels of the spine. Multilevel degenerative changes can result in decreased mobility of the spine and even fusion between the intervertebral bodies. Disc herniation, especially when painful, also results in reduced mobility and diminished levels of activity. These chronic changes associated with degenerative changes and disc herniation can have profound effects on the sensitive structures within the spinal canal and the spinal musculature.

SPINAL STENOSIS

The expansion of the facet joints as a result of degenerative changes can encroach on the central canal and the lateral foramina. This encroachment can

Figure 5.1 Spinal stenosis due to chronic degeneration

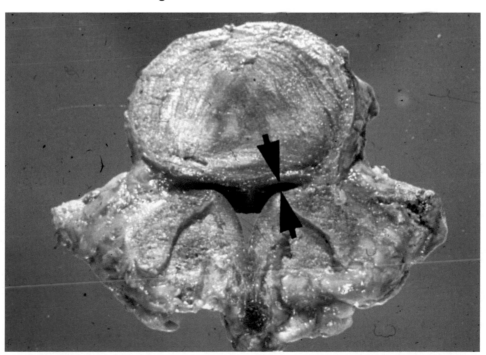

This transverse section of L5 shows marked stenosis of both the central canal and the lateral recesses due to osteophytic growth of the posterior facets and the vertebral endplates. Courtesy Churchill-Livingstone (Saunders) Press

Figure 5.2 Advanced degeneration and bony fusion

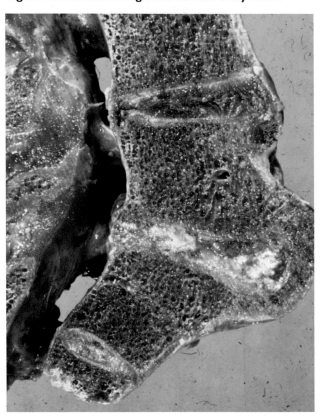

Longitudinal section through the lumbar spine shows marked degeneration and fusion of the bodies of L4–L5 and L5–S1. There is stenosis or narrowing of the central canal at both levels due to osteophytes protruding into the canal at the level of the disc. Courtesy Churchill-Livingstone (Saunders) Press

Figure 5.3 Central stenosis

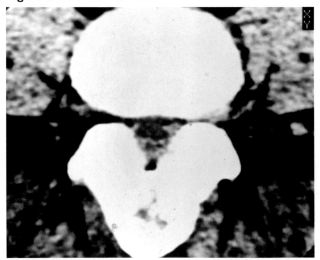

This CT transverse section through the lumbar spine shows marked central canal stenosis. The posterior muscle has been partially replaced by fibrofatty tissue. Courtesy Churchill-Livingstone (Saunders) Press

Figure 5.4 Central canal stenosis

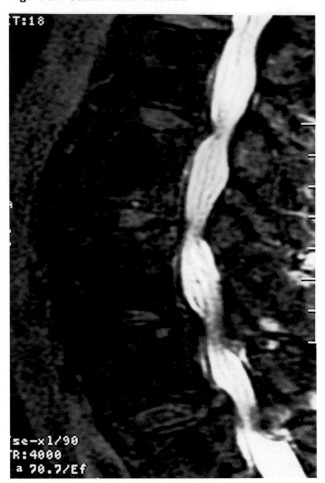

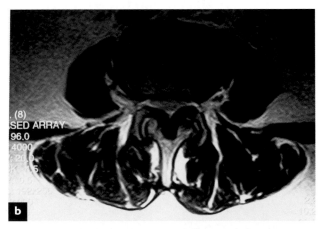

T2 weighted MR sagittal image of the lumbar spine (a), demonstrating high-grade spinal stenosis at L2–L3, L3–L4 and L4–L5. The spinal fluid has a bright signal intensity and the compression of the intrathecal rootlets is apparent. On the axial T2 MR image (b), the central canal stenosis is caused by thickening of the posterior neural arch and ligamentum flavum, and overgrowth of the posterior facet joints. This causes significant flattening of the normally ovoid-appearing thecal sac

Figure 5.5 Multiple-level degenerative lumbar spondylosis and spinal stenosis

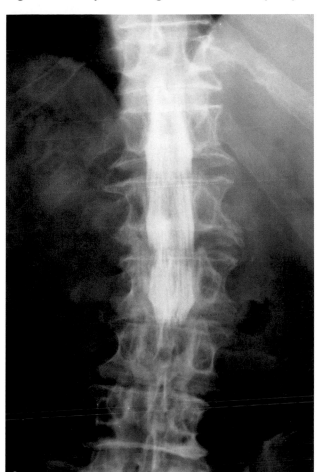

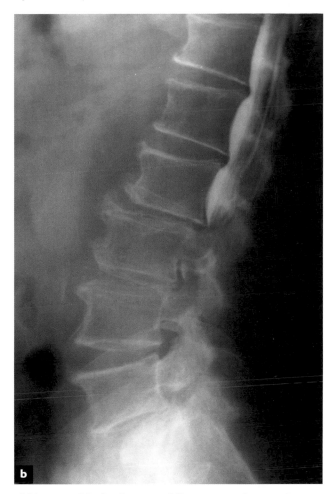

These images are from the same patient. Anteroposterior (a) and lateral (b) views of the lumbar spine following a myelogram, demonstrating a complete block of the contrast at the L2–L3 level

Continued

become quite marked, especially in the presence of large osteophytes from the vertebral bodies, and can result in significant stenosis of the central canal and lateral foramina. These changes can be visualized on MRI and CT scanning, and, when severe, can disrupt function within the spinal cord and nerve roots. Such disruption can be intermittent and associated with pain or numbness in the legs on activity and which is relieved with rest, known as neurogenic claudication, or it can become permanent, leading to neurologic deficits as a result of encroachment on the spinal cord or cauda equina.

The degree of spinal stenosis can be measured on CT and MRI imaging. Hypertrophy of the posterior facets encroaching on the neuroforamen is also evident in this type of study. The effect of compression on the spinal cord, cauda equina and/or nerve roots is determined by electrodiagnostic studies.

MUSCLE TRAUMA, IMMOBILIZATION AND ATROPHY

As degenerative changes progress in the spine or following disc herniation, the mobility of the spine is greatly reduced and patient activity is limited as a result of pain. This immobilization has profound effects on paraspinal muscles. Within 3–4 weeks, atrophy of the muscle fibers can be seen on microscopy. The cells become smaller, the number of nuclei decreases and the spaces between muscle fibers increase in size. Within 7 weeks, the spaces between muscle fibers become large and filled with fibrous collagen and the degeneration of muscle fibers becomes prominent. During exercise and remobilization of the spine, regeneration can be seen in the muscle fibers. Prominent myoblast chains are formed centrally in the empty sheath of damaged

Figure 5.5 *continued* **Multiple-level degenerative lumbar spondylosis and spinal stenosis**

These images are from the same patient. Intrathecally enhanced axial computed tomogram reveals central canal stenosis secondary to posterior facet joint hypertrophy and vertebral body osteophyte formation and disc bulging (c). Sagittal proton density MR image (d) demonstrates multiple level spondylotic changes and central canal stenosis at L2–L3 and L3–L4. Axial MR image (e) reveals central canal stenosis

Figure 5.6 Electrodiagnostic studies in spinal cord injury

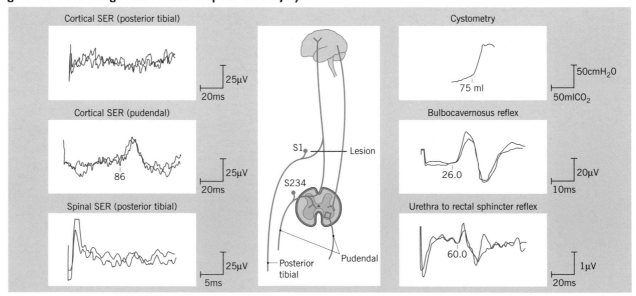

Somatosensory evoked responses from the posterior tibial and pudendal nerves are blocked as they travel through the spinal cord. The reflex studies from the bulbocavernosus and urethra to the rectal sphincter are intact below the level of the injury. Cystometrogram shows hyperreflexia. The spinal cord injury could be due to fracture, severe central stenosis or tumor encroaching on the neural canal

Figure 5.7 Lumbar disc protrusion

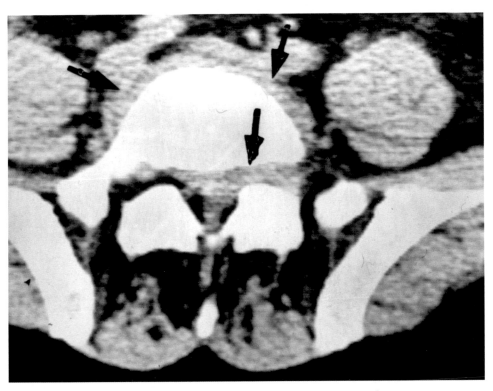

Axial CT image shows a large left-sided disc protrusion (arrow) at the L5–S1 level. The posterior muscle is replaced by fibrofatty tissue due to prolonged inactivity

Figure 5.8 Paraspinal muscle atrophy

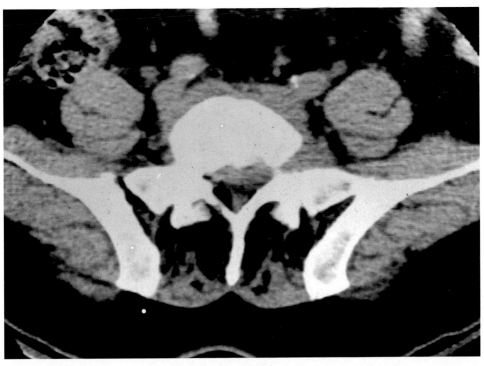

CT axial image of the L5–S1 segment in a patient with a large disc protrusion leading to prolonged inactivity. This has resulted in atrophy and replacement of the posterior musculature with fibrofatty tissue

Figure 5.9 Muscle atrophy at 4 weeks immobilization

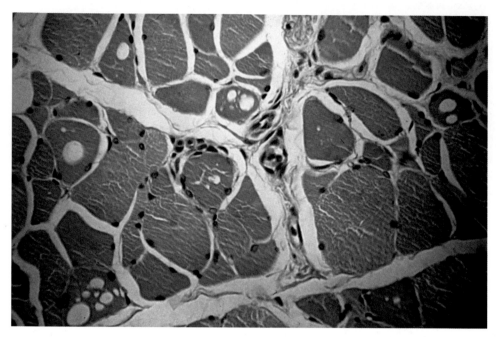

Light microscopy of muscle tissue after 4 weeks of immobilization. The muscle fibers are much smaller than usual and there are a number of empty muscle sheaths. There are empty spaces between muscle fibers and few nuclei in the remaining muscles. Courtesy Churchill-Livingstone (Saunders) Press

Figure 5.10 Muscle atrophy at 7 weeks of immobilization

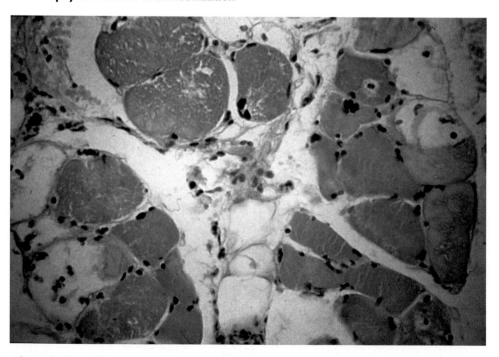

Light microscopy of muscle fibers following 7 weeks of immobilization. Note the larger spaces between muscle fibers, sparse nuclei and empty muscle sheaths. Courtesy Churchill-Livingstone (Saunders) Press

Figure 5.11 Muscle regeneration

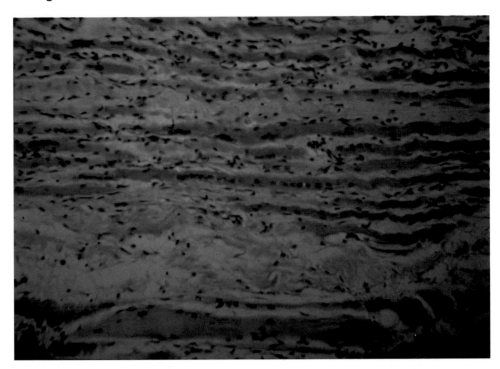

Light microscopy of muscle fibers (human) showing regeneration. There is extensive replacement of muscle fibers with fibrous tissue. There are multiple thin myoblastic chains and muscle fibers with prominent central myoblastic nuclei. Courtesy Churchill-Livingstone (Saunders) Press

Figure 5.12 Muscle regeneration after direct trauma

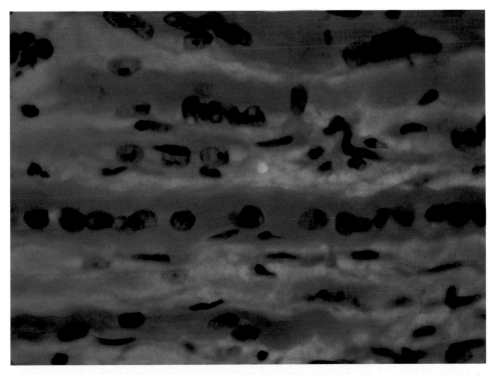

Light microscopy of muscle fibers (monkey) showing regeneration after direct trauma. The transverse band of myoblast nuclei is noted to be central in a new muscle fiber. Courtesy Churchill-Livingstone (Saunders) Press

Figure 5.13 Muscle regeneration

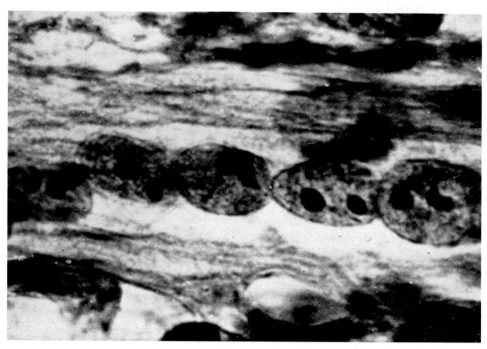

Light microscopy of muscle (cat) showing muscle regeneration. There is a central band of myoblast nuclei, each with two small dark nucleoli. Courtesy Churchill-Livingstone (Saunders) Press

Figure 5.14 Muscle 3 months after injury

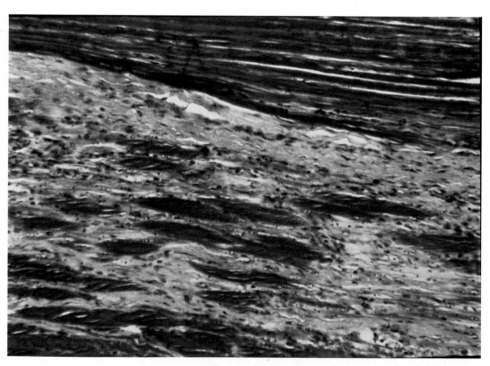

Light microscopy of muscle (monkey) 3 months after injury. The upper field shows new muscle fibers (red). The lower field shows primarily collagen (yellow) with a few muscle fibers (red). Courtesy Churchill-Livingstone (Saunders) Press

Figure 5.15 Muscle 3 months after injury

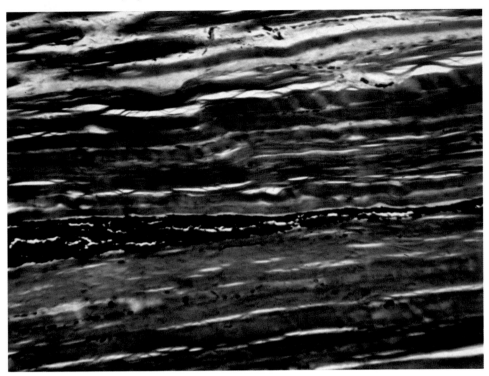

Light microscopy, longitudinal section of muscle fibers (monkey) 3 months after direct injury. There is a full field of new thin muscle fibers. Courtesy Churchill-Livingstone (Saunders) Press

Figure 5.16 Muscle atrophy, electron microscopy

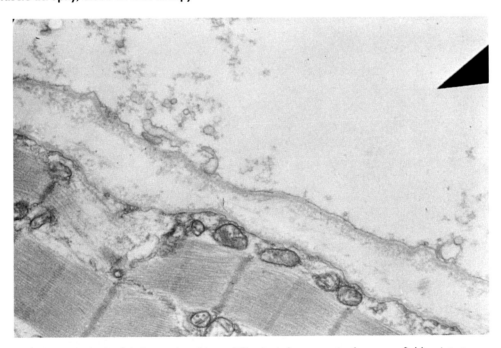

Electron microscopy of muscle (cat) after 3 months of immobilization; the arrow in the upper field points to a completely empty sarcolemmal sheath. In the lower field, there are almost normal muscle fibers with visible mitochondria. Courtesy Churchill-Livingstone (Saunders) Press

Figure 5.17 Muscle regeneration, electron microscopy

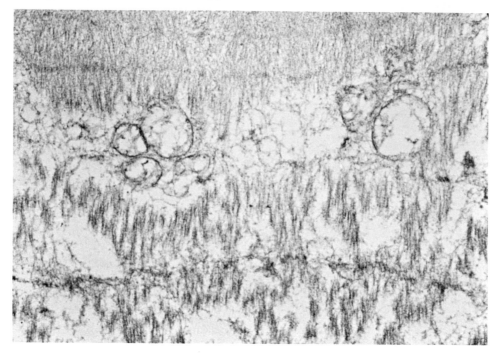

Electron microscopy of muscle (cat) 2 months after immobilization. There is degeneration of muscle with a few transverse Z-lines in a sea of debris. Courtesy Churchill-Livingstone (Saunders) Press

Figure 5.18 Muscle regeneration, electron microscopy

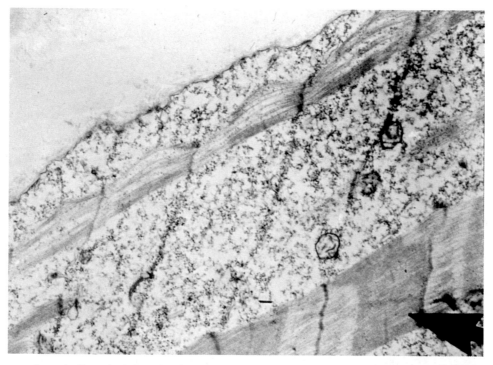

Electron microscopy of muscle fibers (cat) 4 weeks after activity is renewed following a period of inactivity. The regeneration process can be seen in the development of new Z-lines. The arrow points to a new fiber. Courtesy Churchill-Livingstone (Saunders) Press

Figure 5.19 Muscle regeneration, electron microscopy

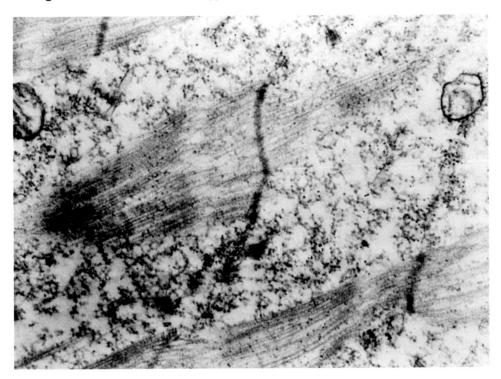

Electron microscopy of muscle (cat) showing regeneration. There are two new vertical Z-lines and a few transverse muscle filaments. Courtesy Churchill-Livingstone (Saunders) Press

Figure 5.20 Muscle regeneration, electron microscopy

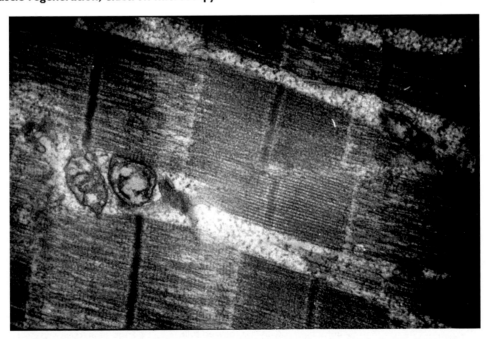

Electron microscopy of muscle (cat) 3 months after renewed activity following a period of immobilization. The muscles have regenerated fully. Note the mitochondria on the left of the field. Courtesy Churchill-Livingstone (Saunders) Press

muscle fiber and the amount of actin and myocin increases. The Z-lines begin to re-form and the nuclei migrate to the periphery of the fiber.

On CT and MR imaging of the spine, it is possible to visualize these changes within the posterior musculature. With immobilization, the posterior muscles are gradually replaced by fibrofatty tissue which increases with prolonged periods of inactivity.

BIBLIOGRAPHY

Cooper RR. Alterations during immobilization and regeneration of skeletal muscle. *J Bone Joint Surg* 1972;54A:919

Kirkaldy-Willis WH, McIvor GWD. *Spinal Stenosis. Clinical Orthopaedics and Related Research.* Philadelphia: JB Lippincott 1976;115:114

6

Spinal deformity

Traumatic, congenital and degenerative changes can all result in deformity of spinal structures. Many of these abnormalities are of no clinical consequence, but under certain circumstances can predispose a patient to increasing pain. Other deformities such as scoliosis can result in cosmetic and functional difficulties.

SPONDYLOLYSIS

The vertebral arch attaches to the vertebral body through the pedicles. The laminae originate from the pedicle at a comparatively weak area known as the pars interarticularis or isthmus. In childhood and adolescence, this area is subject to fatigue fracture, which may not heal properly and can lead to a fibrous union rather than a stable bony union. This can happen unilaterally or bilaterally. If it occurs

Figure 6.1 Spondylolysis

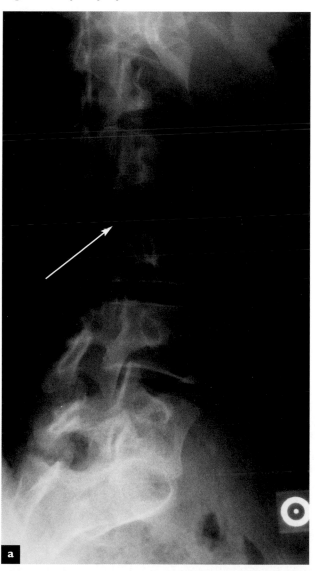

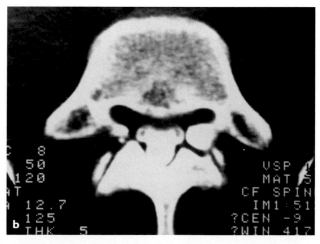

Oblique radiographic view of the lumbar spine with a spondylolysis at L3 (arrow) (a). Axial CT demonstrates the neural arch defect in the pars interarticularis (b)

Figure 6.2 Spondylolytic spondylolisthesis

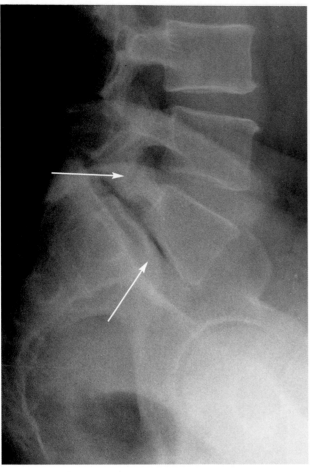

Lateral radiograph of the lumbar spine reveals a spondylolytic spondylolisthesis at L5–S1 (upper arrow). The L5 vertebra has moved forward approximately 50% on S1. The L5 disc space is narrowed, and the Knuttson gas phenomenon is seen in the disc space (lower arrow)

Figure 6.3 Spondylolytic spondylolisthesis

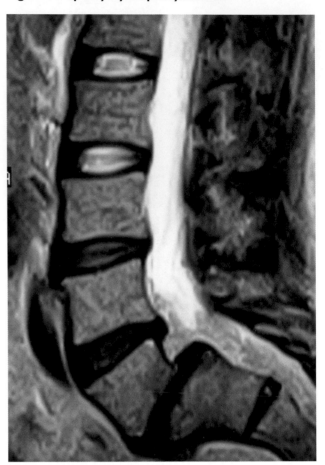

Sagittal T2 weighted magnetic resonance image demonstrates a spondylolytic spondylolisthesis at L5–S1. The L3–L4, L4–L5 and L5–S1 discs all show a diminished signal intensity, indicative of disc degeneration. This patient has a high shear angle at L5–S1, which may predispose to developing a spondylolisthesis. The central spinal canal is not narrowed since the neural arch does not move anteriorly

bilaterally, it creates an area of weakness between the anterior and posterior components of the vertebral arch. If this is stable, it may not be clinically important and can be an incidental finding seen on X-rays and CT scan.

ISTHMIC SPONDYLOLISTHESIS

The weakness caused by a spondylolysis, especially if it is present bilaterally, can cause a separation of the anterior and posterior elements of the vertebral arch. This results in a slippage of the superior vertebral body on the inferior vertebral body. The stress caused by this slippage can result in increased sheer on the disc, which in turn leads to degenerative changes. As the spondylolisthesis progresses, an instability can occur between the two adjacent vertebral segments. This instability adds further stress and may increase the anterior slippage of one vertebra on the other. As this deformity progresses, there is enlargement of the central spinal canal. The increased instability can also lead to disc herniation at the level of the spondylolisthesis. Nerve root irritation can occur as a result of the instability of the motion segment and pseudoarthrosis material that may cause a mass effect that may encroach on the nerve root within the subarticular recess.

Figure 6.4 Segmental instability at L4–L5 secondary to spondylolysis at L4

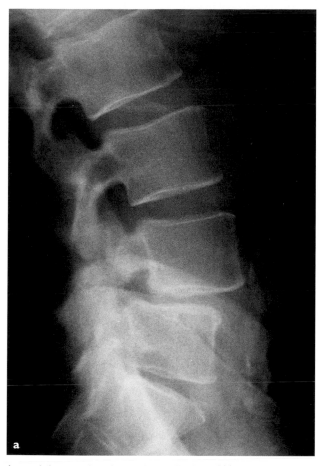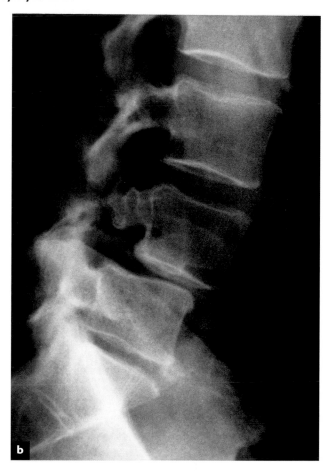

Lateral dynamic bending radiographs (a and b)

Figure 6.5 Isthmic spondylolisthesis

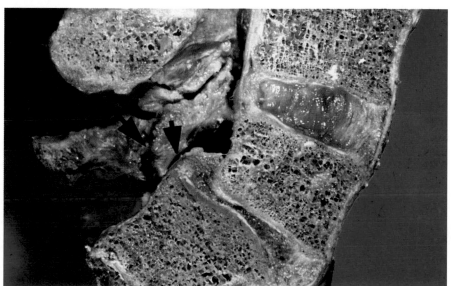

Longitudinal section through the lumbar spine shows an isthmic spondylolisthesis or anterior slippage of L5 on S1. The left arrow points to the defect in the isthmus which allows the slippage to occur. The right arrow points to narrowing of the nerve root canal. There is marked degeneration of the L4–L5 posterior joints and marked loss of the L5–S1 disc substance

DEGENERATIVE SPONDYLOLISTHESIS

During the process of degeneration, there is a period in which the two adjacent segments are hypermobile. The intervertebral disc space becomes narrow and there is laxity and hypermobility of the facet joints. This allows for the anterior displacement of the superior vertebra on the inferior vertebra. This, in turn, can lead to narrowing of the central spinal canal and neurologic deficits. Hypermobility of the facets joint also leads to osteophyte formation and enlargement of the superior articular process of that motion segment, narrowing the subarticular recess and leading to lateral recess stenosis encroaching on the nerve root.

SCOLIOSIS

There are a number of changes in the spine that can result in deformity of the normal vertical alignment of spinal segments. This deformity or scoliosis occurs in both the coronal and sagittal planes. This can occur as a result of congenital defects in the vertebrae as a result of failure of formation and/or segmentation of the vertebra. It can occur spontaneously in adolescence by an undefined mechanism and can progress throughout the adolescent years, causing significant spinal deformity. Scoliosis can also occur as a result of advanced degenerative changes which may be asymmetric, causing the

Figure 6.6 Degenerative spondylolisthesis

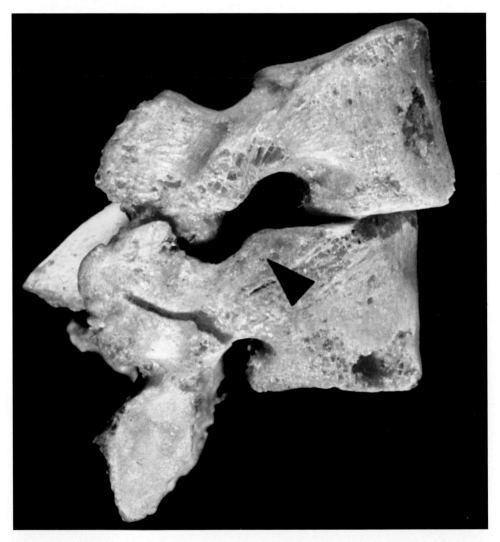

Lateral anatomical specimen shows the displacement of L4–L5 seen in degenerative spondylolisthesis. The L4 nerve can become entrapped posterior to the body of L5 (arrow)

Figure 6.7 Instability due to degeneration of the disc

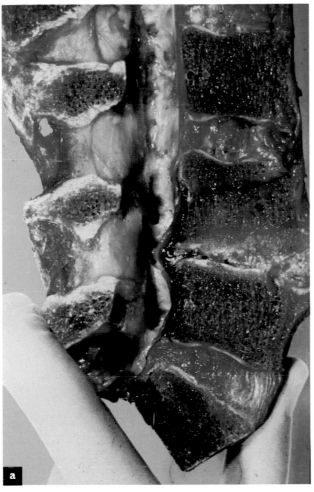 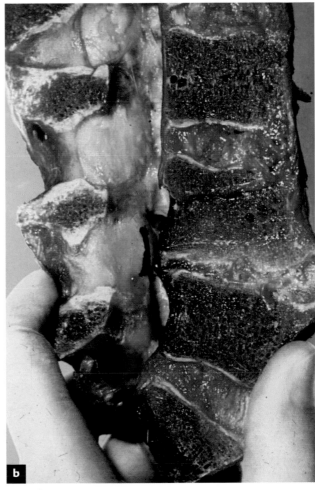

Longitudinal view of the lumbar spine shows extensive degeneration of the L4–L5 intervertebral disc with loss of disc material and narrowing of the disc. This leads to abnormal movement or instability of the segment (a). There is bulging of the annulus at the posterior aspect of the disc, resulting in narrowing of the central canal and foramen. On rotation of the vertebrae, the lateral canal becomes even narrower (b)

vertebrae to rotate and lose their alignment with each other.

INFLAMMATORY DISEASES

There are a number of systemic diseases that impact on the spine and can result in changes in bony structure, resulting in deformity. Rheumatoid arthritis causes laxity in the ligaments, particularly in the cervical spine, and can lead to slippage of one vertebra on the other. Rheumatoid arthritis commonly affects the C1–C2 articulation, but can also affect the subaxial spine. This is usually manifested by spondylolisthesis and instability on flexion and extension lateral radiographs of the cervical spine.

Scheuermann's disease is a condition of unknown etiology whereby there is progressive wedging of vertebrae with the appearance of endplate defects. Material from the intervertebral disc can herniate into the vertebral body, causing multiple level Schmorl's nodes. As this progresses, there is an increase in the normal thoracic kyphosis. In a percentage of patients, this is asymmetric, causing a low degree of lateral scoliosis. Neurologic deficits, however, are unusual in this condition. Paget's disease is another bone disorder that can cause bone deformity. The exact etiology is again not clear, but there is an increase in both the osteoplastic and osteoblastic activity within the bone, resulting in deformity of the structure of the bone.

Figure 6.8 Degenerative spondylolisthesis

Figure 6.9 Congenital scoliosis

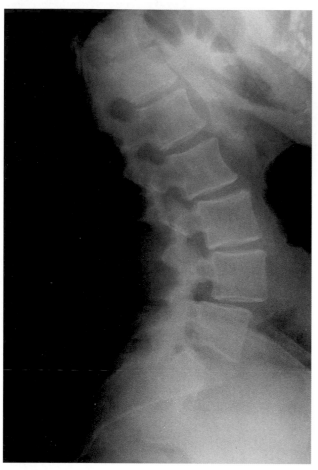

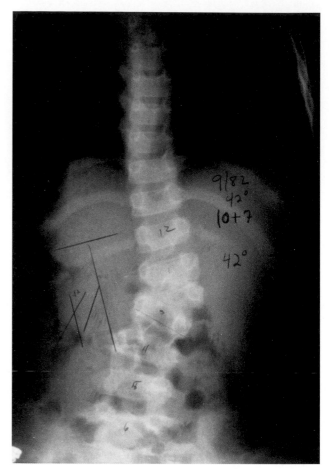

Lateral radiograph of the lumbar spine demonstrates a degenerative spondylolisthesis at L4–L5. When the apophyseal (facet) joints degenerate before the intervertebral disc degenerates, the superior vertebra moves anterior relative to the inferior vertebra. This may cause narrowing of the central spinal canal

Anteroposterior view of the thoracolumbar spine with a 42° curve. The hemivertebra is caused by failure of formation

Figure 6.10 Degenerative lumbar spondylosis and scoliosis

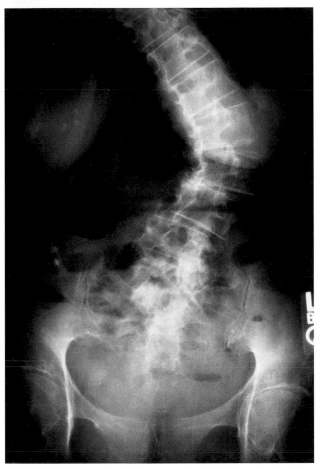

This radiograph shows advanced degenerative changes at multiple levels in the lumbar and lower thoracic spine which have resulted in rotational scoliosis convex to the left side

Figure 6.11 Rheumatoid arthritis of the cervical spine

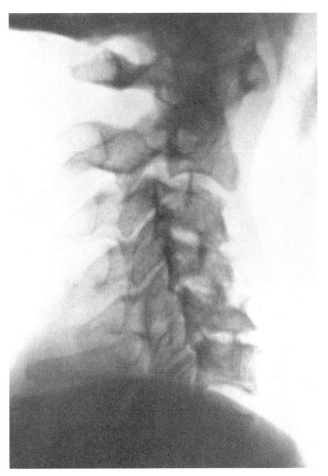

Lateral radiograph shows anterior displacement of C2 on C3. Rheumatoid arthritis may involve the C1–C2 articulation and the subaxial spine, resulting in ligamentous laxity and instability on flexion and extension

Figure 6.12 Paget's disease of the lumbar spine

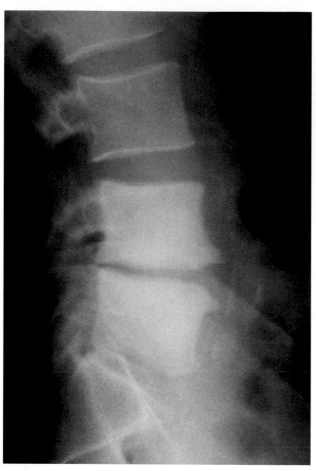

Figure 6.13 Scheuermann's kyphosis

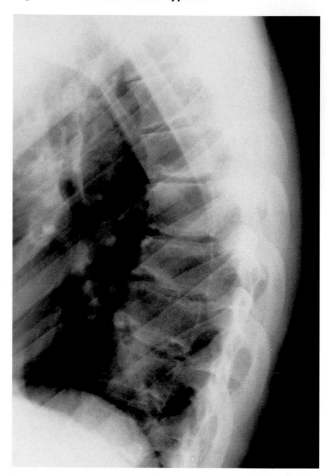

Lateral radiograph demonstrates increased radiodensity in the L4 and L5 vertebrae with narrowing of the disc space and degenerative osteophytes in a patient with Paget's disease of bone

Lateral radiograph of the thoracic spine in a patient with Scheuermann's kyphosis. There is wedging of three adjacent vertebral bodies, and Schmorl's nodes (endplate defects where the disc material herniates into the vertebral body)

BIBLIOGRAPHY

Herkowitz HN, Abraham DJ. Degenerative lumbar spondylolisthesis. *Semin Spine Surg* 1999;11:28

Iqbal MM. Osteoporosis: epidemiology, diagnosis and treatment. *S Med J* 2000;93:2

Kaplan FS, Singer FR. Paget's disease of bone: pathophysiology, diagnosis and management. *J Am Acad Orthopaed Surg* 1995;3:336

Lonstein JE. Natural history and non-operative decision making for adolescent idiopathic scoliosis. *Semin Spine Surg* 1997;9:68

Lucas TS, Einhorn TA. Osteoporosis: the role of the orthopaedist. *J Am Acad Orthopaed Surg* 1993;1:38

Southern EP, An HS. Classification, diagnosis, radiography, natural history, and conservative treatment of spondylolisthesis. *Semin Spine Surg* 1999;11:2

Tribus CB. Scheuermann's kyphosis in adolescents and adults: diagnosis and management. *J Am Acad Orthopaed Surg* 1998;6:36

7

Space-occupying and destructive lesions

Tumors and infections of the spine are much less common than in other organ systems. Primary or metastatic tumors or abscesses affecting the axial skeleton may be expansile and cause mass-effect, compressing neural tissues. These lesions may also cause destruction to adjacent bony structures, rendering the spine unstable and prone to pathological fracture. Although these lesions are rare in the general population of patients suffering from back pain, they are amongst the most serious of the conditions that can present as back pain.

Figure 7.1 Benign tumor

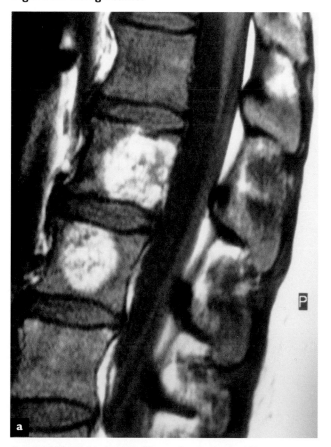 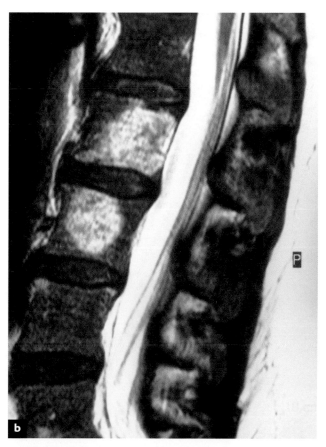

Sagittal MR T1 (a) and T2 (b) weighted images of lumbar spine demonstrate benign hemangiomas in the bodies of L2 and L3. These lesions typically have high signal intensity on both T1 and T2 weighted images. Although benign and usually asymptomatic, when these highly vascular lesions become very large, there is the potential for pathological fracture

Figure 7.2 Osteoid osteoma

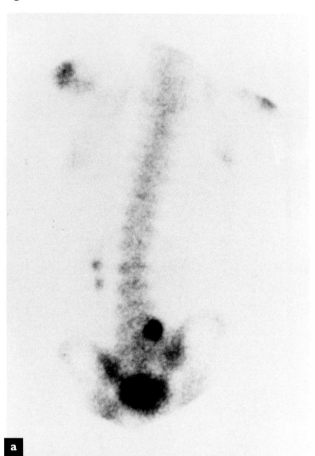

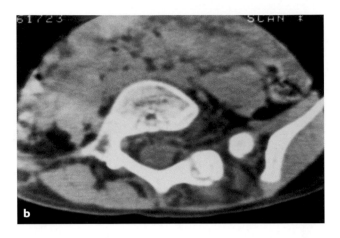

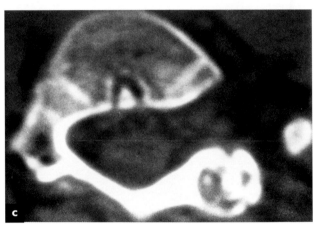

A 6-year-old child with localized back pain and scoliosis. The technetium-99m bone scan demonstrates focal increased uptake of the radiopharmaceutical at L5 (a). Axial CT soft tissue (b) and bone density settings (c) confirm an expansile process in the lamina of L5 on the left with a central nidus. These benign tumors typically produce nocturnal back pain which is relieved by aspirin

SPINAL TUMORS

Tumors that affect the spine can be primary benign or malignant tumors originating in spinal tissues or metastatic tumors spreading from other organs. Benign hemangiomas can be seen in the vertebral bodies on imaging studies and present as incidental areas of high vascularity which tend to be asymptomatic. Although osteoid osteomas do not metastasize, they are nonetheless expansile and tend to destroy bony tissues and encroach on neural elements as they grow. There is often an inflammatory thickening of the bone adjacent to an osteoid osteoma, which can be seen on CT scan, and lights up on technetium bone scans. The malignant tumors such as the sarcomas can expand to a very large size, destroying the bony tissue surrounding them. Primary soft tissue tumors in the breast, lung, thyroid or prostate, as well as other tissues, can metastasize

to the spine, causing rapidly expanding and often multiple fast-growing soft tissue tumors in the spine. These tumors can erode the vertebral body of the pedicles, leading to collapse of the vertebra and paresis. Multiple myeloma originating in the spine can also lead to destruction of the vertebral body and collapse of the vertebra. If this occurs in the neck, quadriparesis can result.

SPINAL INFECTIONS

Bacterial infections can spread systemically to the spine as part of a generalized infectious process or can be introduced locally following invasive procedures such as discography or surgery. Disc infection following discography leads to the destruction of the disc and the erosion of the adjacent bones. This can result in abscess formation which may encroach on

Figure 7.3 Osteoid osteoma

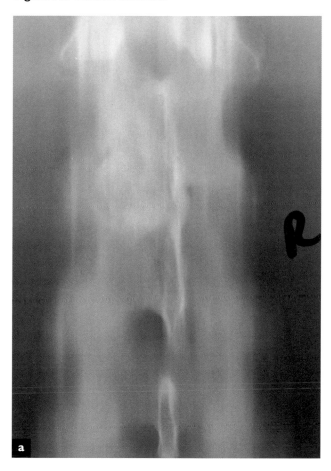

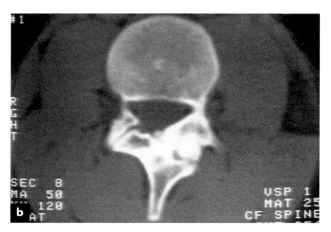

Anteroposterior plain radiographic tomogram of the lumbar spine demonstrates a radiodensity in the left L3 neural arch (a). Axial computed tomogram demonstrates thickening of the L3 neural arch and a lesion with a central nidus (b)

the neural elements. If allowed to progress, vertebral osteomyelitis commonly occurs with further destruction and collapse of the vertebral body. Tuberculosis of the spine and paraspinal tissues is not very common in developed nations, but remains a substantial cause of spinal pain and deformity in certain countries with limited medical facilities. Tubercular lesions can result in abscess formation and reactive changes within bones and ligaments. They can slowly erode the bony structures, leading to collapse of the vertebral body anteriorly with resulting deformity and posterior gibbus formation and often require surgical stabilization.

ARACHNOIDITIS

Inflammation within the arachnoid and subarachnoid spaces can lead to scar formation which can result in clumping and adhesions between the intrathecal rootlets, leading to compression of the nerve roots within the cauda equina. Although not strictly an expansile lesion, arachnoiditis is often associated with inflammatory changes and can result in neural deficits and chronic back pain. The most common cause of arachnoiditis in the past was the injection of oil-based contrast media into the subarachnoid space during myelography. The use of water-based contrast media has substantially reduced the amount of arachnoiditis from myelography. Today, scarring in the perineural structures is more commonly the result of surgical intervention and the healing process that occurs following surgery. Arachnoiditis can also occur as a result of meningitis and other inflammatory conditions of the meninges.

Figure 7.4 Sacral chordoma

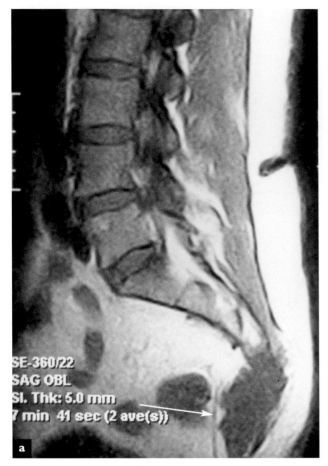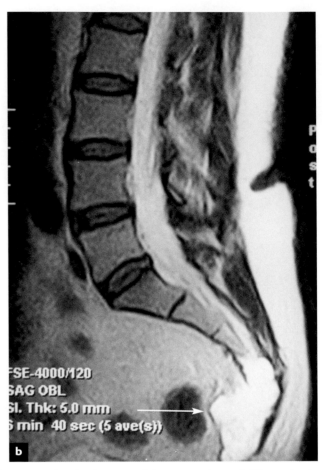

Sagittal MR T1 (a) and T2 (b) images demonstrate a large expansile mass at the distal aspect of the sacrum (arrow). These slowly growing malignant lesions are derived from embryonic notochord cells. Surgical treatment requires a large marginal resection that often necessitates sacrificing sacral nerves, leading to bowel and bladder incontinence

Figure 7.5 Metastatic lesion

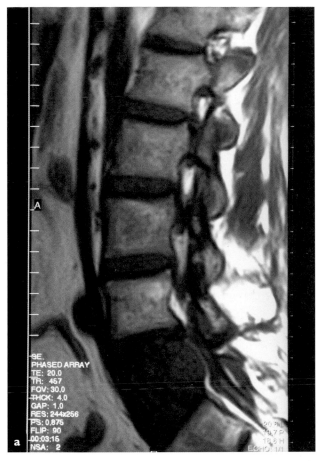

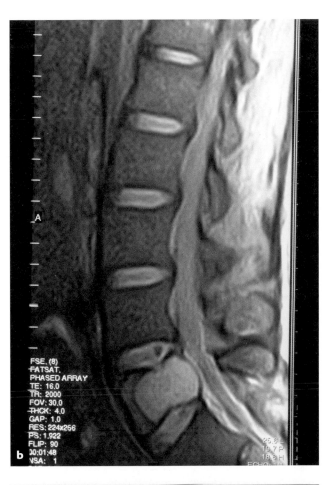

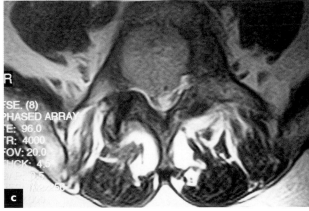

Sagittal MR T1 (a) weighted image and proton density (b) image of metastatic lung carcinoma to the L5 vertebral body. The axial image demonstrates extension of the tumor into the spinal canal, displacing the thecal sac (c). Once a metastatic lesion involves more that 50% of the vertebral body, there is an impending risk of pathological fracture

Figure 7.6 Metastatic lesion

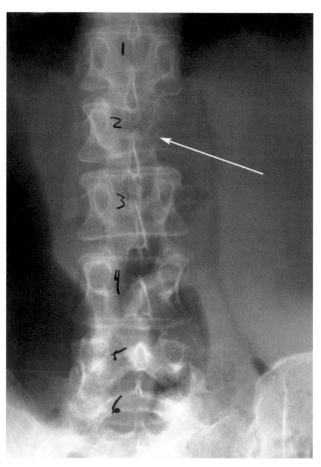

Anteroposterior view of lumbar spine in a patient with a metastatic lesion to the L2 vertebra. The so-called 'winking owl' sign is seen (arrow). Radiographic involvement of the posterior neural arch and pedicles is a pathognomonic sign of metastasis

Figure 7.7 Lymphoma

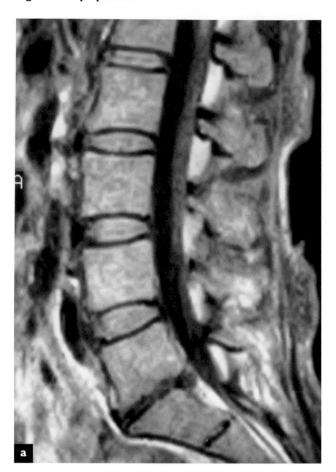

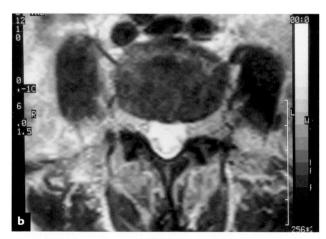

T1 weighted sagittal (a) and T2 axial (b) MR image of a patient with lymphoma. Note the mottled appearance of the marrow. Diffuse osteopenia, multiple myeloma, and systemic marrow replacement diseases will give an abnormal marrow appearance. MR imaging utilizing spin echo T1, proton density, and T2 sequences, as well as fat suppression and gadolinium enhancement techniques, are useful diagnostic features of MRI when evaluating bone marrow diseases

Figure 7.8 Myeloma

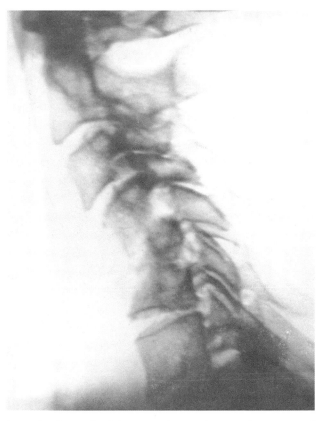

Lateral radiograph of the cervical spine showing destruction of the mid-cervical vertebral bodies. This type of lesion destroys the vertebral bodies and can lead to compression fractures and deformity

Figure 7.9 Discitis and vertebral osteomyelitis

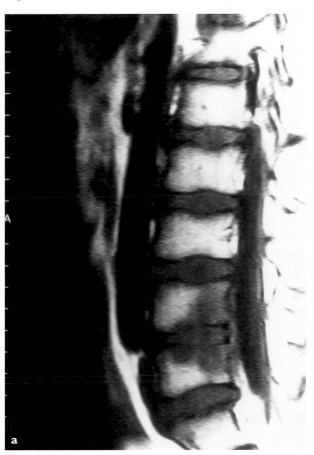

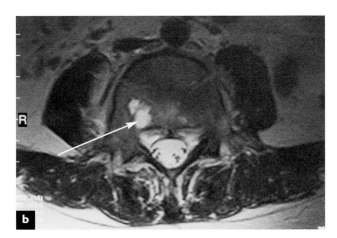

Sagittal MRI demonstrates decreased signal intensity in the adjacent L4 and L5 vertebrae (a). Aspiration of the L4–L5 disc space was positive for *Staphylococcus aureus*. The axial image (b) demonstrates a high signal intensity region on the right side of the vertebral body which is indicative of an active pyogenic process (arrow)

Figure 7.10 Discitis following discography

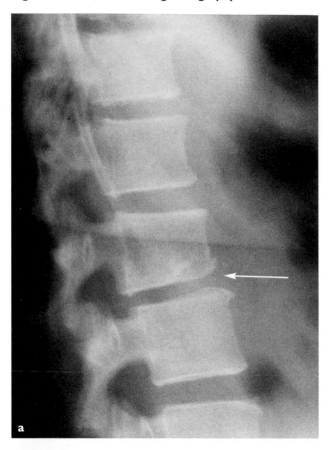

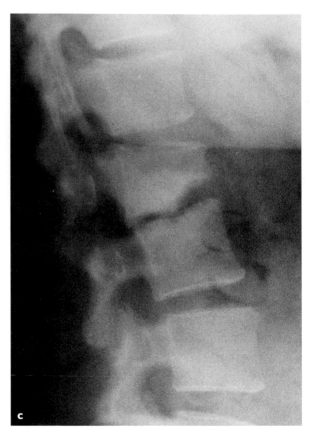

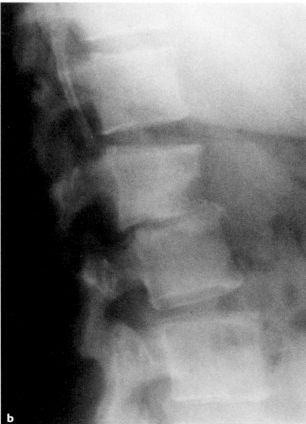

Lateral radiograph of lumbar spine 3 weeks after lumbar discography shows an area of radiolucency in the anterior inferior aspect of the L3 vertebra (arrow) (a). At 6 weeks, there is interspace collapse and mild retrolisthesis of L3 on L4 (b). The disc space aspiration cultured *Escherichia coli*. The same patient is shown at 6 months (c)

Figure 7.11 Osteomyelitis of the thoracic spine

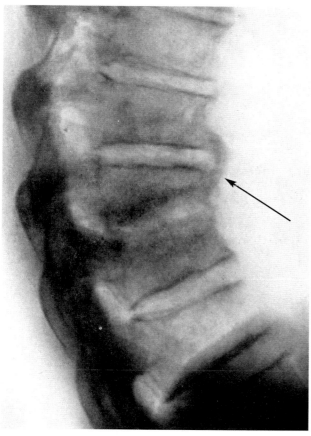

Staphylococcus aureus infections of the spine ae not uncommon. Drug addiction and AIDS are predisposing causes. Abscesses in the vertebral body, new bone formation and sclerotic changes are common. Destructive lesions leading to collapse of the vertebral bodies are rare in this type of infection

Figure 7.12 Tuberculosis of the thoracic spine

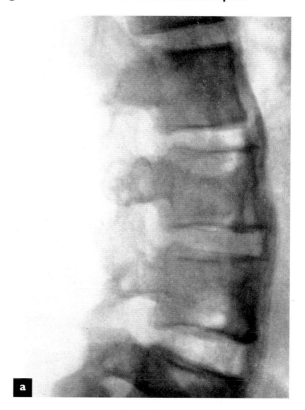

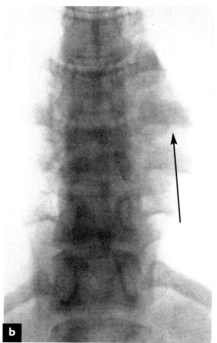

Inflammation caused by the tubercle bacillus rarely causes ossification of the anterior common ligament. Paraspinal abscesses are commonly encountered. Destruction of an intervertebral disc and of adjacent vertebral body bone is common in neglected cases. In such cases, spinal fusion, preferably anterior, with intervertebral interbody bone grafts is often required, especially in the third world

Figure 7.13 Tuberculosis of the cervical spine

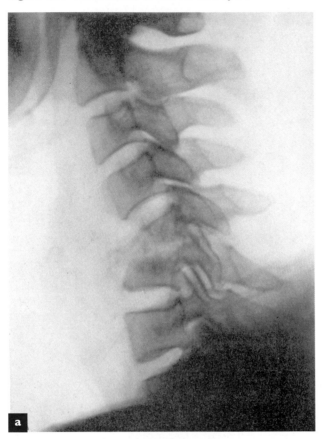

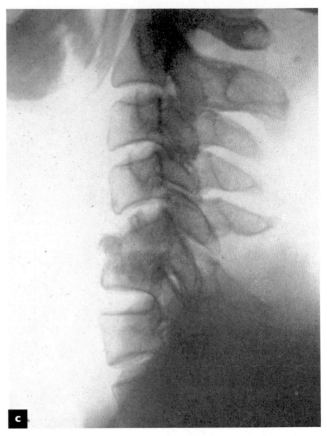

(a) Destruction of the cervical vertebral bodies by tuberculosis leads to anterior collapse as seen in these lateral radiographs. (b) The vertebrae can be approached surgically from the front. (c) Fusion of the vertebrae is usually evident on radiographs 3 months following surgery

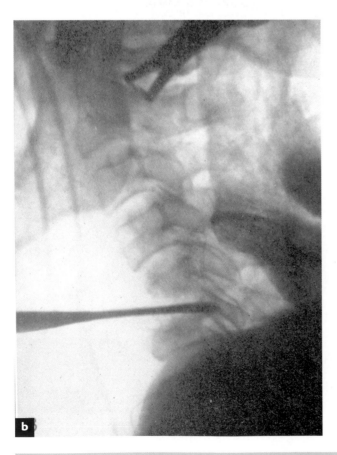

Figure 7.14 Tuberculosis of the lumbar spine

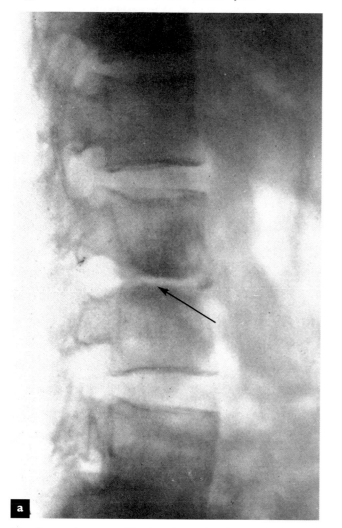

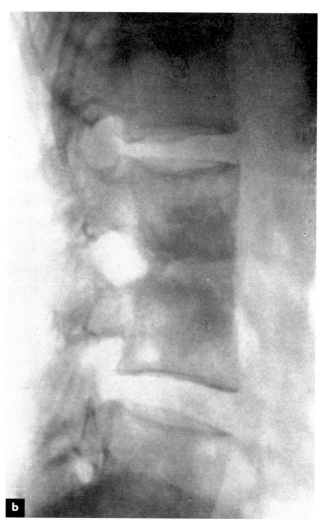

The destruction caused by the tubercle bacillus can lead to instability (a) that may be stabilized by surgical fusion (b) as seen in these lateral radiographs

Figure 7.15 Tuberculosis of the lumbar spine

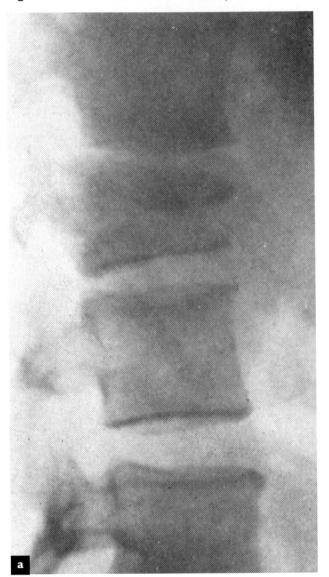

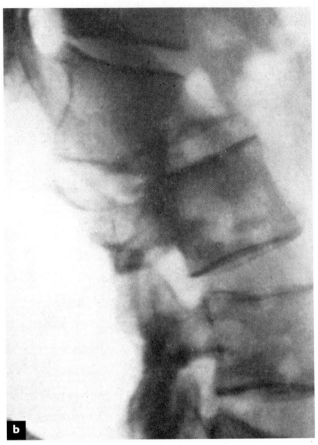

Surgery does not always stop the progression of the tuberculous process. If stability cannot be achieved by surgical fusion, then the vertebrae may collapse and displace with marked deformity that may lead to paraplegia

Figure 7.16 Brucellosis of the lumbar spine

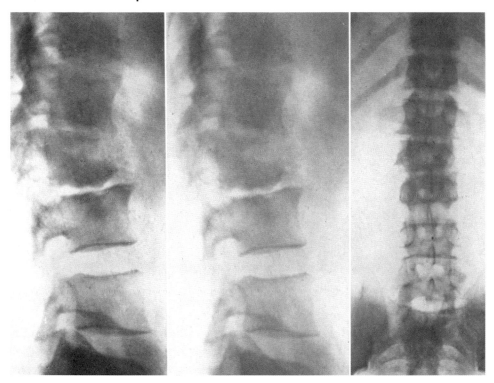

This is uncommon but calls for consideration in making a differential diagnosis. It is often caught from infected cattle. It is characterized by a combination of new bone formation and erosion of bone

Figure 7.17 Pseudomeningocele

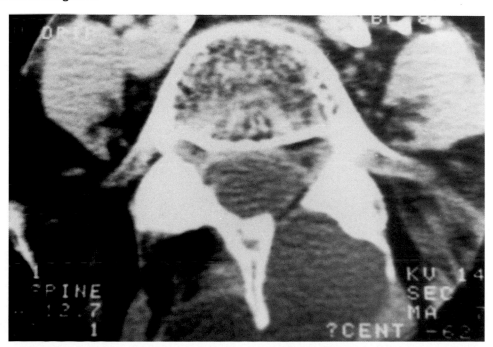

This postoperative CT at L4–L5 reveals a laminotomy defect on the left side and a large fluid-filled mass which is in continuity with the thecal sac. The fluid signal density is the same as that of cerebrospinal fluid. Small pseudomeningoceles are usually asymptomatic and require no treatment. Larger ones may cause back pain and headaches, which may be reproduced by direct pressure over the cutaneous level of the lesion

Figure 7.18 Adhesive arachnoiditis

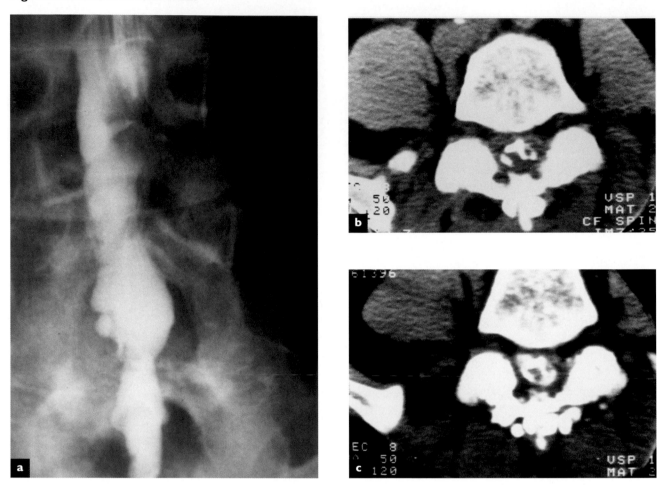

This patient had undergone multiple myelographic studies using oil-based contrast media as well as five surgical procedures to the lumbar spine. The anteroposterior myelographic view using water-soluble contrast reveals distortion of the thecal sac (a). The non-enhanced axial CT demonstrates calcific arachnoiditis at L4–L5 (b). The intrathecally enhanced CT at the same level reveals clumping of the nerve rootlets (c)

BIBLIOGRAPHY

Dagirmanjian A, Schils J, McHenry M, Modic M. Spinal osteomyelitis. *Semin Spine Surg* 1997;9:38

Khan I, Vaccaro AR, Zlotolow DA. Management of vertebral diskitis and osteomyelitis. *Orthopaedics* 1999; 22:758

8

Spinal surgery

Many of the destructive and compression lesions in the spine, including disc herniations, spondylolisthesis, spinal tumors, spinal fractures and spinal infections, may require surgical intervention to stabilize the spine or remove the neural compressive lesion. In recent years, there has been a rapid expansion in the number and complexity of available surgical options. The surgical techniques can be divided into three basic categories.

The first includes the minimally invasive techniques in which the vertebral structure being operated on is approached using either needles or catheters to inject proteolytic chemicals into the disc, steroids or analgesics into the facets and paraspinal soft tissue structures, or a thermal needle into the disc to ablate the discal tissues. These methods, however, can only be used in well-localized lesions that can be accessed percutaneously.

The second approach is surgical decompression. This is the more common procedure, as many lesions of the lumbar spine require removal of a mass lesion, such as a disc protrusion, tumor or abscess, through a surgical incision. This requires dissection of the skin and musculature to reach the lesion, followed by the surgical removal of the offending lesion. The spinal structures can be approached surgically from the back through the posterior spinal musculature, through the ribcage via a flank incision, or anteriorly through the neck or abdomen.

The third category of surgical procedures are those which attempt to reduce mobility in the spine by fusing two or more segments. Such fusion can be achieved by approaching the spine either posteriorly or anteriorly. The surgeon may elect to place cortical or cancellous bone grafts across two or more vertebrae in order to create a bony fusion through

Figure 8.1 Posterior fusion of the lumbar spine

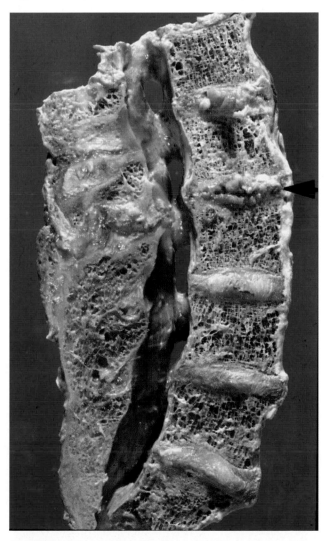

Longitudinal section through the lumbar spine shows surgical bone graft fusion of the posterior elements of L3 to the sacrum, with narrowing of the L2–L3 disc and canal at this level due to new bone formation above the fusion

Figure 8.2 Surgical approach to the cervical spine

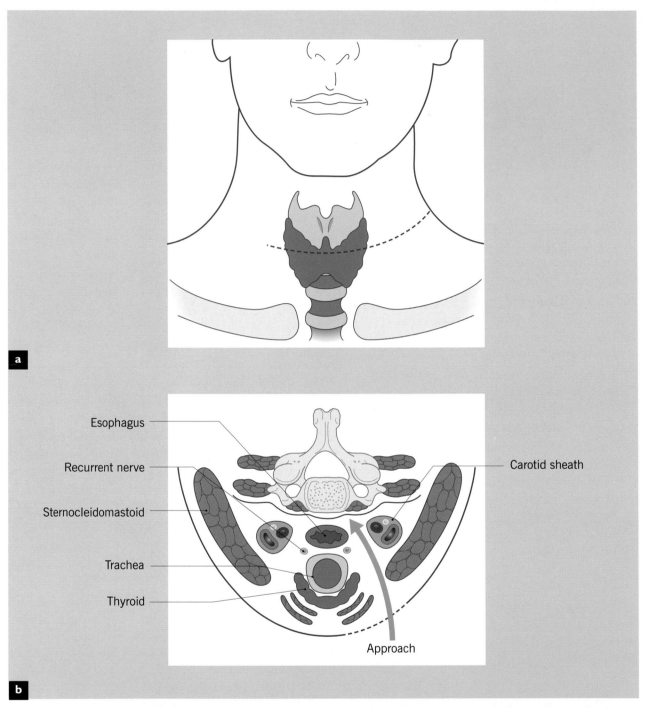

Esophagus

Recurrent nerve

Sternocleidomastoid

Carotid sheath

Trachea

Thyroid

Approach

(a) The incision is made anteriorly at the level of the trachea (C4–C6); (b) the cervical spine is visualized by separating the soft tissues and retracting the thyroid gland to one side (arrow)

the normal healing process. Alternatively, the surgeon may elect to place a metal stabilizing device through the pedicles of adjacent vertebra, locking them together, or remove the offending disc and place one of a number of sophisticated metal devices or bone within the disc space to maintain separation between the vertebral bodies and allowing for fusion. Fusion of multiple segments, however, increases the sheer forces on the joint above the fusion and can lead to degenerative changes and instability at levels above and below the fusion.

Figure 8.3 Anterior cervical fusion

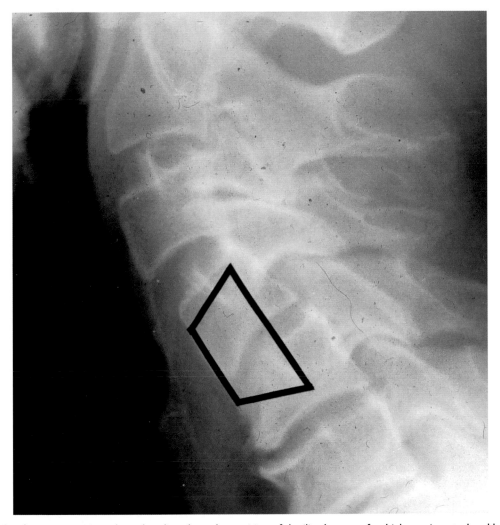

The dark lines that form a trapezium-shaped outline show the position of the iliac bone graft which was inserted and locked into position in slots cut in the bodies of the 4th and 5th cervical vertebrae. The vertebral bodies of C4–C5 show complete union of the bones. There are degenerative changes in the form of narrowing of the disc space and osteophyte formation. The fusion is thought to present additional stressors on adjacent vertebrae which can aggravate the degenerative changes

Figure 8.4 Anterior spinal fusion at L5–S1 using a bone dowel

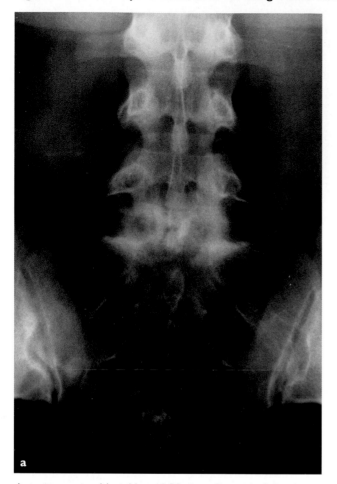 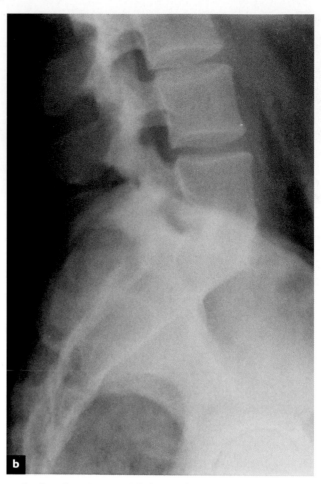

Anteroposterior (a) and lateral (b) views 5 months following an anterior lumbar discectomy at L5–S1 and fusion utilizing autogenous iliac crest bone graft and allograft threaded bone dowels

Figure 8.5 Anterior interbody fusion at L5–S1 using a titanium cage

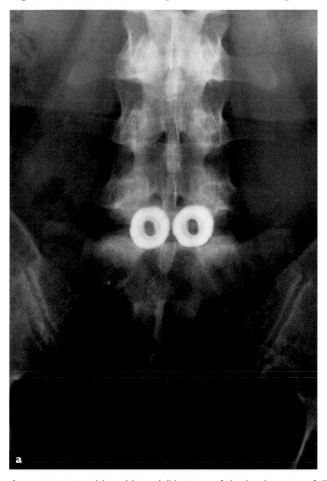 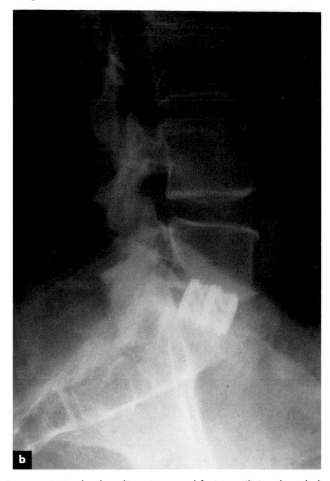

Anteroposterior (a) and lateral (b) views of the lumbar spine following an anterior lumbar discectomy and fusion, utilizing threaded cages filled with autogenous iliac crest bone graft

Figure 8.6 Posterior fusion at L5–S1 using pedicle screw fixation

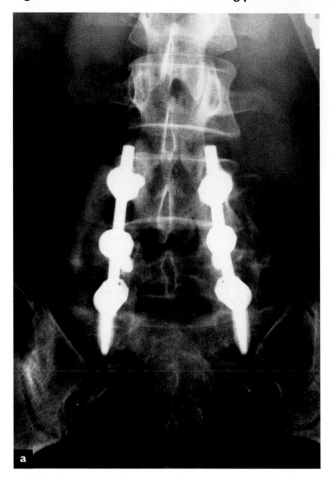 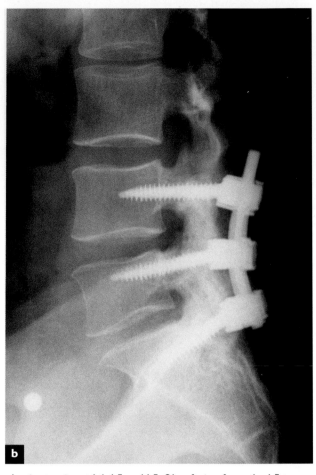

Anteroposterior (a) and lateral (b) views of the lumbar spine following laminotomies at L4–L5 and L5–S1, a fusion from the L5 transverse process to the ala of the sacrum

Figure 8.7 Posterior fusion of the lumbar spine using iliac crest bone grafts

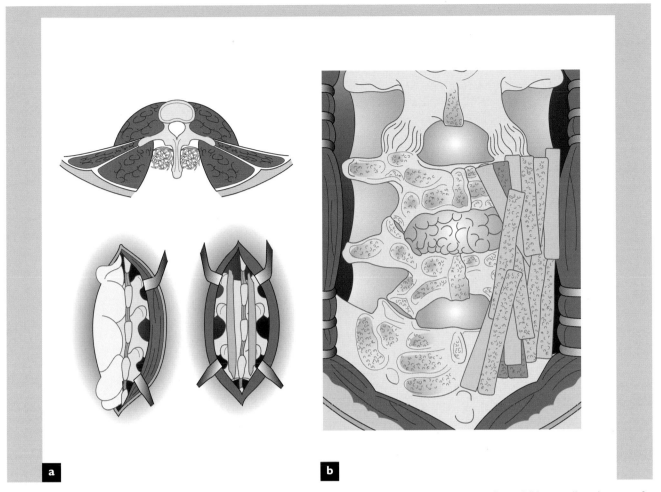

These figures demonstrate the method of fusing the lumbar spine posteriorly using (a) twin tibial grafts and (b) cancellous bone grafts harvested from the iliac crest

Figure 8.8 Anterior fusion of the upper thoracic spine

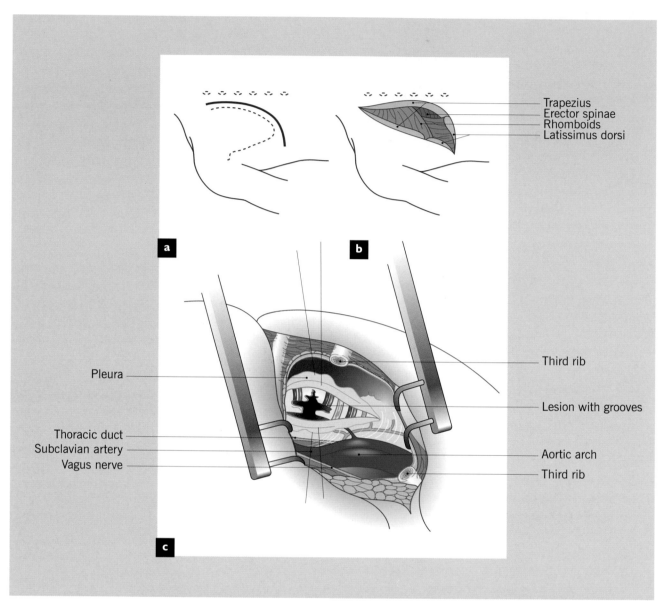

(a) The curved paravertebral incision is made medial to the scapula; (b) the third rib is removed; (c) the pleura is then incised to allow visualization of the upper thoracic spine

Figure 8.9 Anterior fusion of the mid-thoracic spine

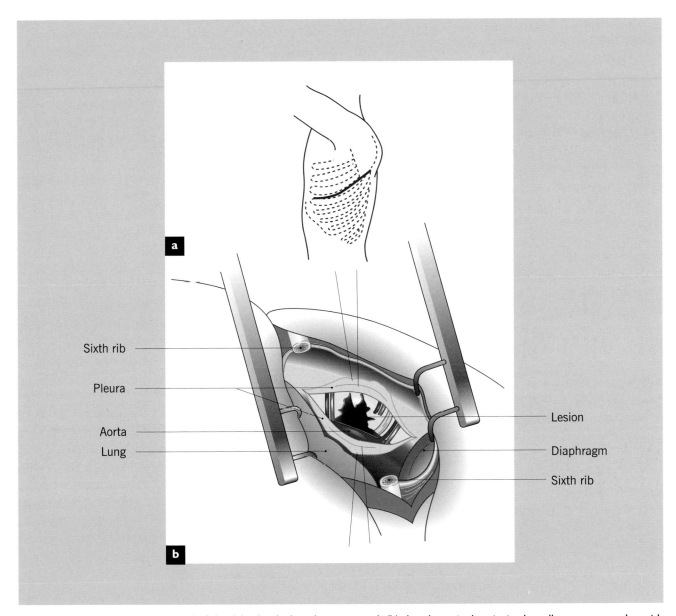

Sixth rib

Pleura

Aorta

Lung

Lesion

Diaphragm

Sixth rib

(a) The incision is made at the level of the 6th rib which is then removed; (b) the pleura is then incised to allow access to the mid-thoracic spine

Figure 8.10 Anterior fusion of the lower thoracic spine

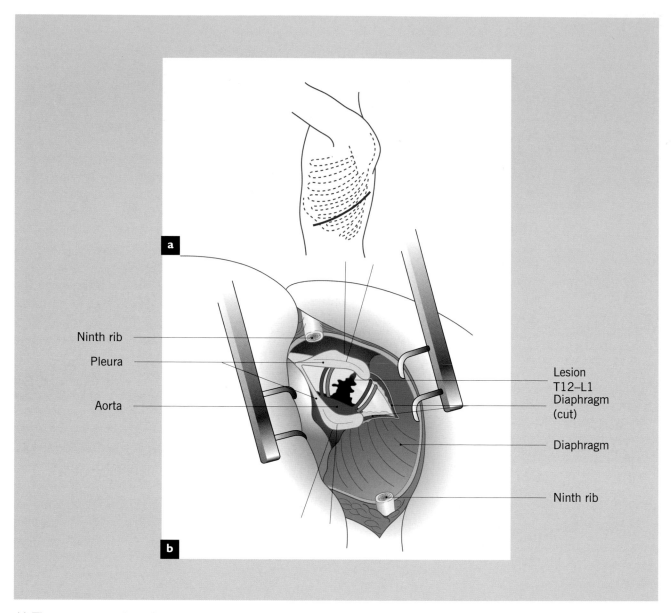

Ninth rib

Pleura

Aorta

Lesion
T12–L1
Diaphragm
(cut)

Diaphragm

Ninth rib

(a) The incision is made at the level of the ninth rib which is removed; (b) the posterior diaphragm is divided to give access to the lower thoracic spine

Figure 8.11 Oblique lateral approach to the anterior lumbar spine

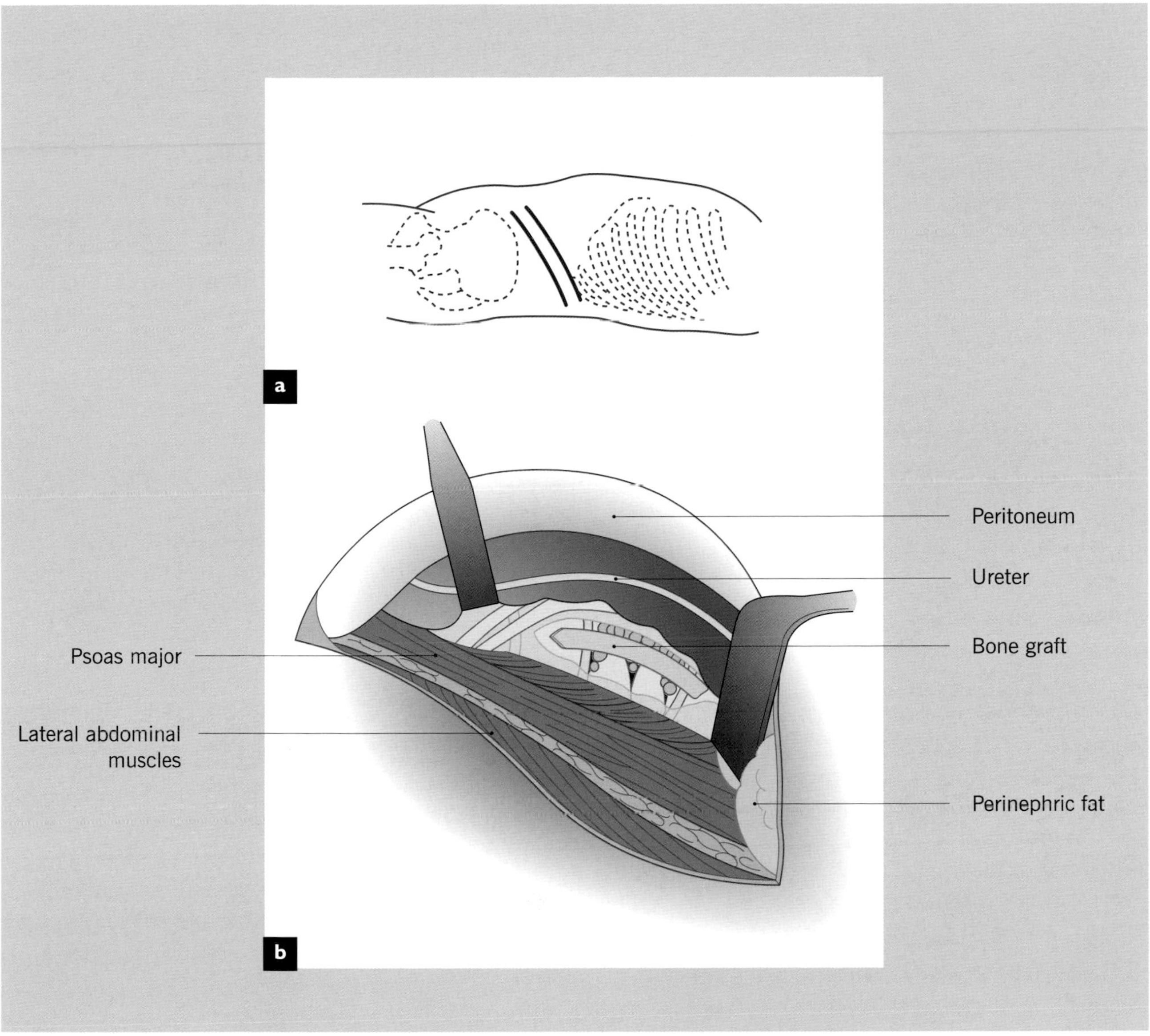

Peritoneum

Ureter

Bone graft

Psoas major

Lateral abdominal muscles

Perinephric fat

(a) The lumbar spine is approached posteriorally; the parallel dark lines represent two different skin incisions. (b) The peritoneum and contents are retracted forward to expose the lumbar spine, care being taken not to injure the ureter. The peritoneum is not opened

Figure 8.12 Anterior approach to the lumbo-sacral spine

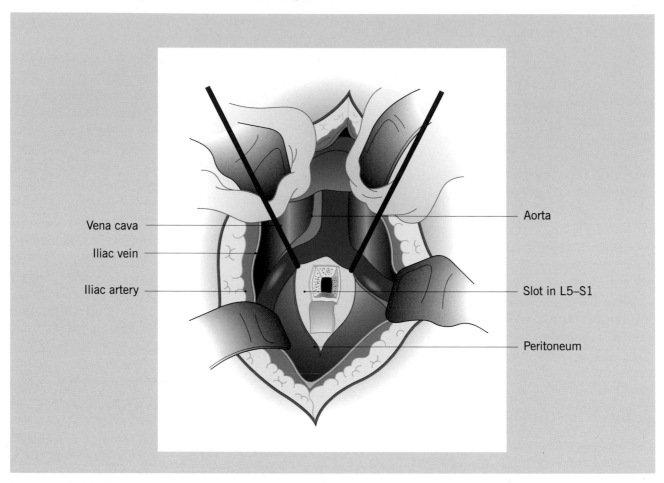

Vena cava

Iliac vein

Iliac artery

Aorta

Slot in L5–S1

Peritoneum

Lesions at the L5–S1 level may be approached through an anterior mid-line abdominal incision. The peritoneum is opened and the bowel is retracted to expose the lumbo-sacral junction. Bone is removed to create a slot crossing the body of L5 and the upper part of the sacrum. A bone graft can then be wedged into the slot to create a one-level anterior fusion

Figure 8.13 Costotransversectomy

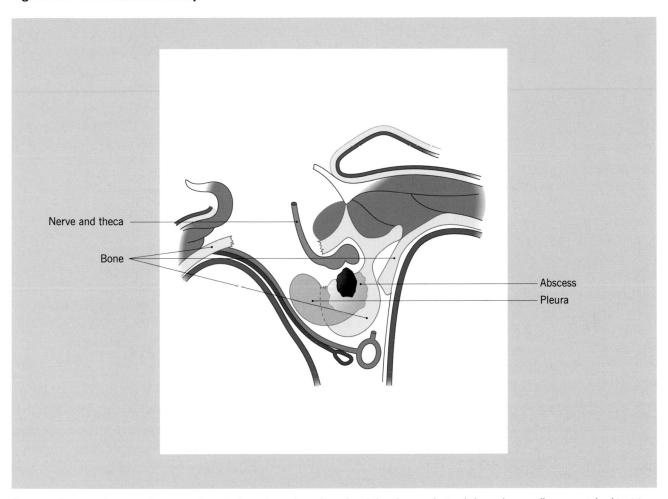

Pressure from an abscess adjacent to the spinal cord may be relieved and the abscess drained through a small paravertebral incision. A transverse process and 2 inches of the posterior part of the rib at the level of the lesion are removed. The abscess and one black-colored sequestrum are shown here in cross-section before removal

Figure 8.14 Antero-lateral decompression of the thoracic spine for Pott's paralysis

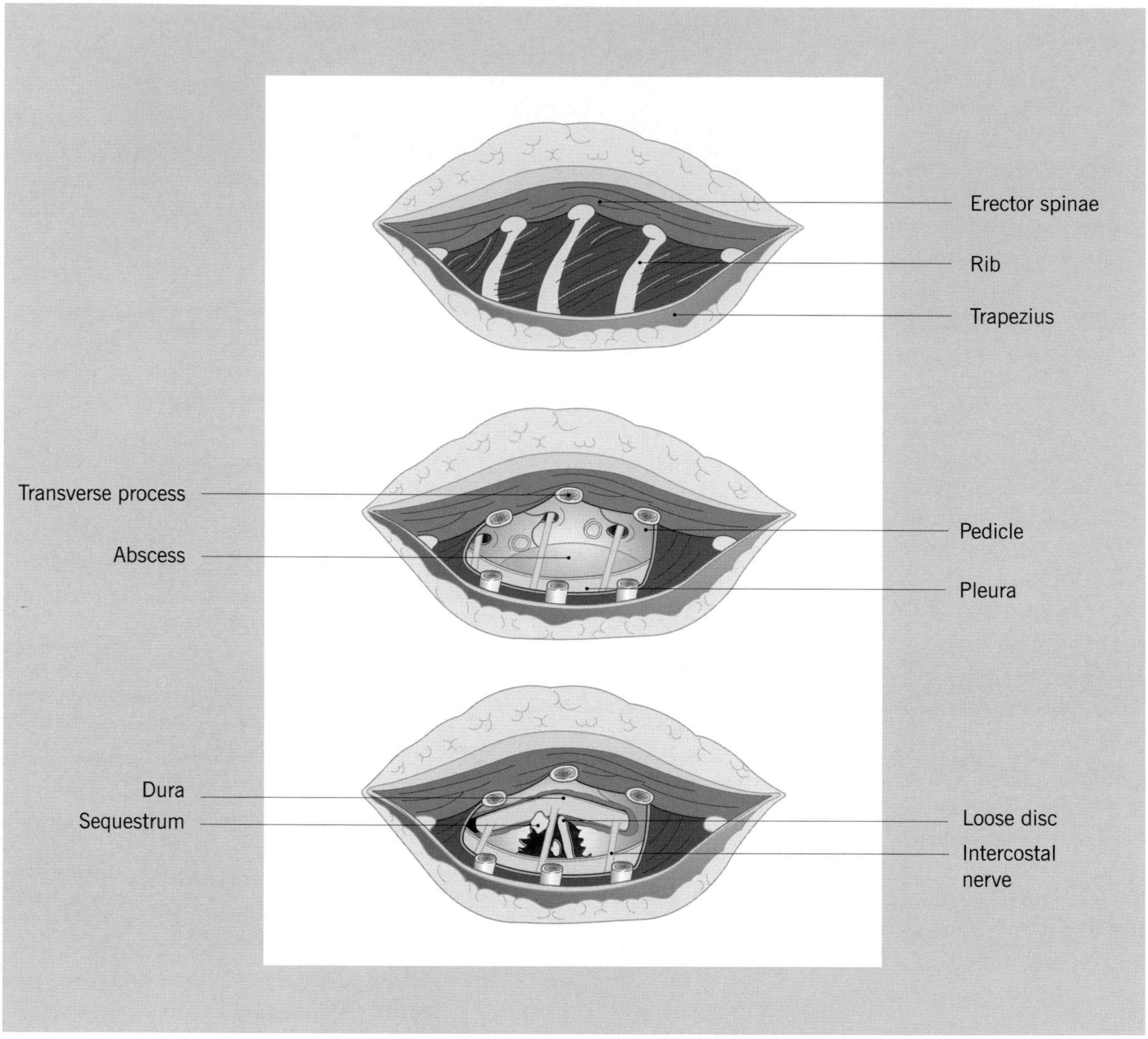

Erector spinae

Rib

Trapezius

Transverse process

Abscess

Pedicle

Pleura

Dura

Sequestrum

Loose disc

Intercostal nerve

This approach is employed in cases of Pott's paraplegia when an abscess is causing direct pressure on the spinal cord and direct access to the dura is essential. (a) Exposure of 4–5 inches of the posterior part of three ribs centered over the lesion; (b) exposure and removal of the visible portions of the ribs expose the lateral aspect of the vertebral bodies; (c) a lateral window has been cut in the vertebral bodies, crossing the disc space and lesion and exposing the dura. This permits removal of pus, granulation tissue, sequestrum and bony ridges pressing on the spinal cord

BIBLIOGRAPHY

Dirksmeier PJ, Parsons IM, Kang JD. Microendoscopic and open laminotomy and discectomy in lumbar disc disease. *Semin Spine Surg* 1999;11:138

Kirkaldy-Willis WH, Wood AM. *Principles of the Treatment of Trauma.* Edinburgh: E. and S. Livingstone, 1962:223–37

Roaf R, Kirkaldy-Willis WH, Cathro AJ. *Surgical Treatment of Bone and Joint Tuberculosis.* Edinburgh: E. and S. Livingstone, 1959

Truumees E, Sidhu K, Fischgrund JS. Indications for fusion in lumbar disc disease. *Semin Spine Surg* 1999;11:147

Vaccaro AR, Ball ST. Indications for instrumentation in degenerative lumbar spinal disorders. *Orthopaedics* 2000;23:260

9

Selected bibliography

Frymoyer JW, ed. *The Adult Spine. Principles and Practice*, 2nd edn. Philadelphia: Lippincott-Raven, 1997

Haldeman S, ed. *Low Back Pain. Neurology Clinics*. Philadelphia: WB Saunders, 1999

Kirkaldy-Willis WH, Bernard TN, eds. *Managing Low Back Pain*, 4th edn. London: Churchill Livingstone, 1999

Wall PD, Melzack R. *Textbook of Pain*, 4th edn. London: Churchill Livingstone, 1999

White AH, Schofferman JA, eds. *Spine Care*. St Louis: Mosby Year-Book Inc., 1995

Index

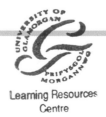